Before this story begins, the inside cover of this book is designed to create a safe space for calm reflection.

This beach scene and beautiful jacaranda tree, to me, represent a place of love, memory, calm and return.

Not all landscapes in life, or in this book, are literal. Some exist purely to hold what words cannot.

TESTIMONIALS

When Jodi asked me to review her memoir, I felt deeply honoured. Having had the great fortune of getting to know her many years ago, her joyfulness, intelligence, ability to love deeply and her hard-earned wisdom have been a source of inspiration and encouragement ever since. Naturally, I was eager to read her memoir – to see her life unfold from her own perspective. And the book didn't just meet my expectations – it exceeded them.

Jodi's voice throughout her memoir feels completely authentic and unguarded. She doesn't shy away from the darkness – she writes with honesty about her great achievements despite her very challenging start in life but even more so about her lowest points, her vulnerabilities and the rawness of her pain. That candidness makes her story so very human and so relatable. In sharing her story with such honesty and heart, Jodi offers more than just a memoir – she offers solace, inspiration and a reminder that second chances are possible.

For me, it was a moving, beautiful read, a reminder that pain doesn't have to define us, a powerful testament to resilience, love (between people and also dogs!) and healing. If you're drawn to real-life stories of pain and recovery, of struggle and renewal – this one will stay with you.

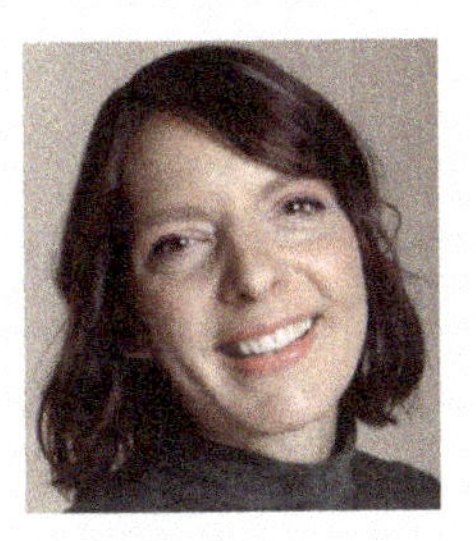

Nele Dumpert,
Fachärztin für
Frauenheilkunde
und Geburtshilfe
OBGYN

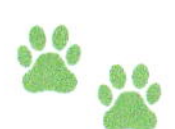

Being an obsessive reader of every genre, I approached Jodi's book *Benni* with healthy scepticism – was this to be another tale of misfortune, self-discovery and recovery? The answer is a resounding "NO". From the outset, I found myself mesmerised, not only at the unbelievable saga of trauma, which, in itself, made for page turning amazement, but at the realisation that each step in Jodi's life to date has been a vital ingredient in her pathway to self-acceptance, self-love and ultimately fulfilment. The title *Benni* seems somewhat perplexing until the latter part of the book. Benni is not only an essential character, but she is symbolic of the path to recovery and finding life's meaning in what can only be described as a circuitous and tortuous road.

Jodi's writing is extraordinarily transparent, giving the reader a rare and honest insight into her very soul, even when delving into her often tragic but ultimately joyful life. She does not shy away from negative appraisals of her journey. I often cried, but not from sadness. I laughed, but not from amusement. I was often perplexed, as to how one person's strength and resilience could evolve so completely. And finally, I rejoiced and experienced true awe of Jodi's continuing compassion, ability to love and forgive others – and herself.

I met Jodi when I was training in obstetrics at a relatively advanced age. Jodi, despite her own massive challenges, mentored and encouraged me to keep going, in the face of what I personally experienced in my professional life as bullying, ageism, overwhelming feelings of inadequacy, imposter syndrome and misogyny. Her positivity and words of wisdom inspired me and have become some of my mantras in my now successful career. I still recall her words: "How you deal with a woman's pregnancy loss will affect her until the day she dies." I take this compassion with me every day, and it has made me a better doctor.

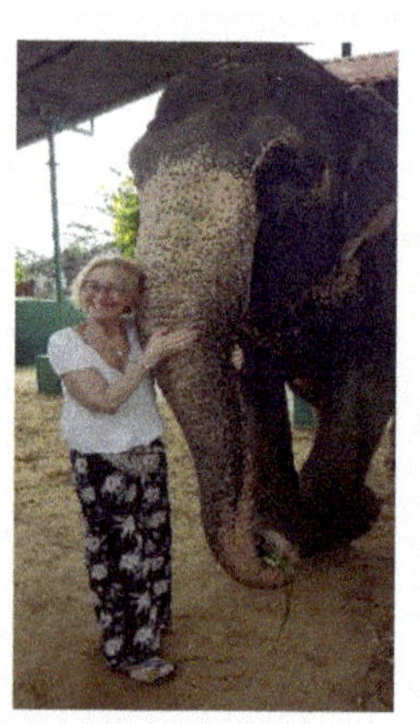

Dr Vivienne Tudeschi
MBBS (hons),
CWH, DRANZCOG
Advanced

Jodi's wonderful book helps one to heal from trauma and find inner peace. Jodi – and Benni – have altered my view of life, relationships and even death in a positive way. You, the reader, will never be quite the same person again.

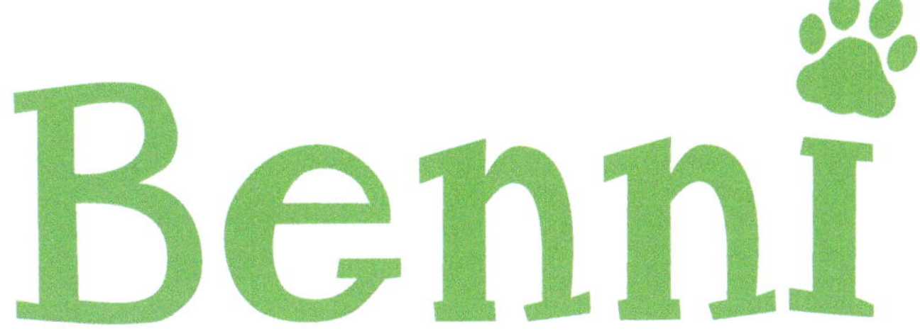

The best medicine has paws

DR JODI-MAREE CRONIN

Benni: The best medicine has paws

ABN: 51647681767
https://dogz4life.com.au
jodi@dogz4life.com.au
Facebook https://facebook.com/dogz4lifeaus
Instagram @benni_the_gsp

This memoir is a recounting of personal experiences and memories as perceived and remembered by the author. Names, dates and details have been changed at times to protect the privacy of some individuals. While every effort has been made to present an authentic portrayal of events, emotions and relationships, it is important to note that memory is fallible and subjective. Dialogues and interactions are based on the author's recollection and may not be verbatim.

Published by Jodi-Maree Cronin.
Cover photo by Empire Art Photography.
Feature illustrations by Cara Ord Create.
Publishing support from Ignite & Write Publishing.

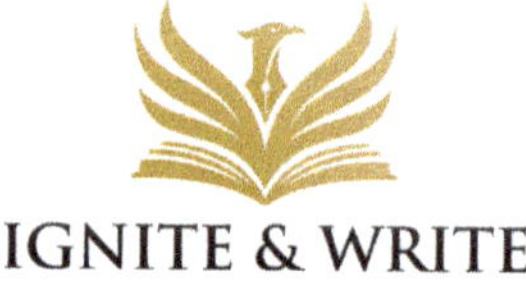

ISBN: Paperback: 978-1-7643724-2-8
Ebook: 978-1-7643724-3-5

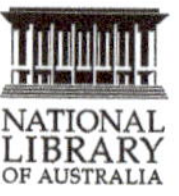

A catalogue record for this book is available from the National Library of Australia

Disclaimer

This book contains content that addresses traumatic events, including but not limited to violence, accidents, loss and other distressing experiences. It may include descriptions or discussions of events that could be triggering for individuals who have experienced trauma or are sensitive to such topics.

The information provided in this book is intended to provide insight, awareness and support for those affected by traumatic events. However, it is not a substitute for professional therapy or counselling. While the author is a registered counsellor, they are not a licensed therapist/psychologist and the content is based on personal experiences, research and general knowledge.

If you are struggling with the effects of trauma, it is important to seek help from a qualified therapist, counsellor or support organisation. You deserve support, understanding and healing, and there are resources available to assist you in coping with traumatic experiences.

- Lifeline (crisis support 24/7): call 13 11 14 or text 0477 13 11 14 for immediate support
- Beyond Blue (support for depression and anxiety): call 1300 22 4636 24/7 or chat online
- Suicide (prevention) 24/7 call back service: call 1300 659 467
- MensLine Australia (24/7 support): call 1300 78 99 78
- MindSpot (free online support for anxiety/depression/stress): call 1800 614 434
- FriendLine (for people feeling lonely): call 1800 424 287
- 1800RESPECT (24/7 support for people at risk of or experiencing family and domestic violence or sexual assault): call 1800 737 732
- 13YARN (a first nations crisis support line): call 13 92 76

To my mum

LEGACY

Your exit planned in exquisite detail, rivalling
the artwork of your many bruises
This was an aggressive illness, an end that no-one ever really chooses
Your values evident in your final letter, full of compassion and love
In death you've become a muse, an endless
source of encouragement from above
I've done my best to create a legacy worthy of a life well lived
You're an inspiration to me, that's for sure,
anything missed I hope you can forgive
You made this world a better place, your everlasting
support stays with me in all I do
I will miss you forever, Mum, but my work
here is done – this one is for you

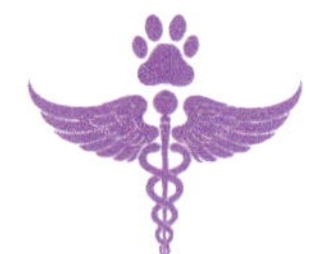

To my baby, Benni

BENNI, THE BEST MEDICINE

Benni, I can't begin to express what you really mean to me
Without your love and support, I'm not sure where I would be
When we met, life had dealt me some very cruel blows
You made me feel better with a simple nudge from your nose
Your antics and sense of humour made training days fun
We surpassed the expectations of absolutely everyone
When health challenged you as much as it did me
We banded together, knowing our relationship was key
With every new challenge, I loved you even more
But not everyone around us could see what we saw
"Thank God for the dog" played over in my mind
How did I get so lucky – you're truly one of a kind
Your name means "blessed" – you brought me back to life
You were just the right medicine I needed to survive

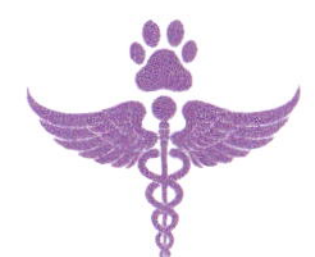

FOREWORD

You are about to read a manual in how the impossible is achievable. I'm not sure if that was Jodi's aim, but here we are.

Looking at her journey to date, it's clear that her path has not been straight and easy, but at every step her determination and defiance of expectation has shone clear.

When we met, I couldn't believe she was married with two small children. Why would someone in our small university in the tropics be juggling a family with study? Surely you go to uni because you've finished school and are trying to avoid the real world a little bit longer. I was barely 17 and had just moved to Townsville, ironically from the same region Jodi and her young family had moved from too. But our experiences were very different. And while I have been aware of that to some degree during our friendship, I hadn't really appreciated it until reading this book. With my perspective as a father of three, I can now see more clearly the sacrifices Jodi and her family were making for her to chase her ambition.

I didn't know this 'mature age student' (not even 23…) was there with focus and motivation that still mystifies me now. All I could see was an incredibly intelligent and driven woman who loved her family in a sincere and protective way. Someone who would refuse to study while her children were awake, who would burn the candle at both ends, and who would take a silly teenage boy to class because he was too dysfunctional to work it out for himself.

Our course was only three years long, but in that time, Jodi became one of my strongest and dearest friends. She moved to Melbourne to continue her studies, while I made my way to Sydney and then back to Queensland. We kept in touch and tried to be there for each other's big career moments. When she found her way back to Queensland, we didn't catch up as frequently as I would have liked. Having a medical career and a young family means there are less gaps in your time for friendships. We always hit full stride as soon as we did catch up though, as if a year's gap had barely been a day. It turns out a lot had been happening in that time, and medicine changes you, sometimes in ways you were expecting, but often catching you unaware and unprepared.

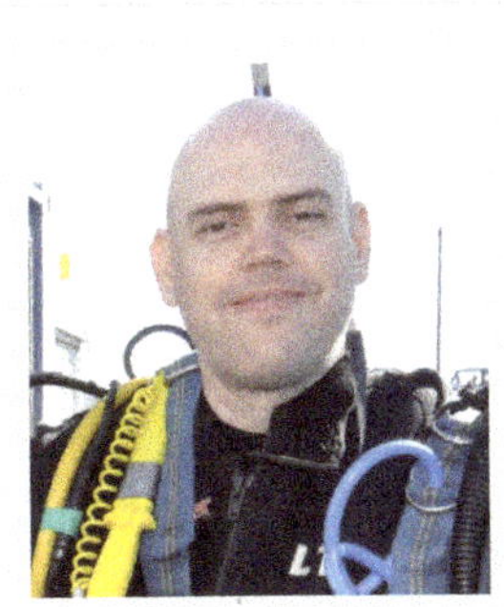

Dr Graeme Kay, B Biomed Sci (Hons), MBBS, FRACGP, Dip DHM (SPUMS)

Jodi has pivoted and learnt to adapt to the unpredictable, finding other avenues of hope and service to the vulnerable. I will never cease to admire her ability to do this.

What this woman has achieved should not be possible, but in doing so she shows us all that no matter the challenge, there is a way to overcome it and continue to shine as a better version tomorrow than we were yesterday.

PROLOGUE

As the traffic around me pulsed like an artery, I felt the hum of the engine, and the air thickened with anxiety with every car that passed by. The world was closing in around me, my heart now pounding so hard in my chest I could hear every beat pumping like heavy metal music in my ears. Even my eyes were pulsating. The car edged ever closer to the massive truck, its engine sending uncomfortable vibrations up to my feet that were almost glued to the floor.

I was far from relaxed, even though I was a passenger. The thick air was making it hard to breathe, my chest was tightening. I felt like I was suffocating. I tried hard to regulate my emotions, but I just couldn't calm my system down. My thoughts were racing, my heart pounding so hard in my chest I wondered if it could be heard from outside my body.

As the car started to overtake, something deep inside me was triggered – this is an old foe, one I know very well and nothing to do with driving capability. I could hear the loud hum of the tyres as the car sped up and my mouth dried up. I could hardly speak but my head was screaming: *No! Don't overtake, I can't handle it.*

"Stop" is the only thing that escaped from my lips as the car started to pull back into the lane, now in front of the giant truck.

It was too late; my system had already reached melting point. It wasn't just fear of the road: it was the echo of another man at the wheel, my father laughing as he swerved towards the edge with a wry grin, yelling, "I'll give you something to be afraid of!" as Mum would beg him to stop and I would squeal out in fear.

He always made it seem like he was just joking. To me, it was a lesson in the abuse of power. Now, decades later, my body remembers. My mind keeps telling me *you're safe* but my body refuses to listen.

PROLOGUE

My body was betraying me in this moment. The overwhelming sense of dread was spreading over me until it reached my head, which began to feel like it was going to explode. Panic set in as my heart pounded like it was about to escape my chest. I knew this feeling well. Serotonin syndrome. *Not again.* I quickly realised this wasn't my normal anxiety. Aware this was chemical and could be dangerous, I said out loud, "I need a doctor." My voice breaking halfway through the sentence.

"Now!" the urgency clear in my voice.

As if heaven sent, there in front of me was the blue and white hospital sign I needed. I gathered all my strength and worked hard on taming the beast, trying to stay alive until I made it safely to the hospital.

Inside the hospital the machines beeped and screamed as if to show my body's distress. My blood pressure was dangerously high, my heart rate was out of control, my temperature rising. As the doctor explained that this was serotonin syndrome again, and could be life-threatening, she quietly warned me, "You need to take this seriously." For the first time, I believed this could end my life.

I called my family, my children, my mum, just in case I didn't make it through the night. In a quiet moment, I thought about the situation I now found myself in. I felt so deeply remorseful. I reasoned: *At least I've had a good life, I know what it feels like to love, to be loved, I hope my babies are taken care of if anything happens to me.*

In that moment I thought: *This is the end.* In a way I guess it was. My life was never going to be the same. The life I had fought so hard to forge could end here, in this sterile little hospital cubicle. My heart still pounding as my world was falling apart.

The hardest part? It was all my fault. There was no-one else to blame, I had done this to myself. I'm the one who tried to end it all.

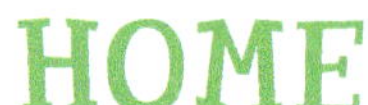

*"**H**ome is where the heart is" you so often hear people say*
***O**thers know that home can be anywhere, even far away*
***M**y home is my haven, a place where I'm most at peace*
***E**veryone's different but for me, home should be where tensions release*

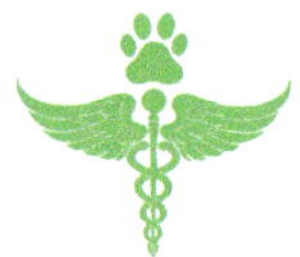

1

My earliest memory is a very vivid one. I'm in a yard, but I can't tell if it's the front or backyard. It's next to a house and there's a concrete strip along which I'm pushing my little three-wheel trike. It's a sunny, moderate day and I'm aware that something really important is going on, but not entirely sure what it is. Mum is at the other end of this concrete strip, talking to someone. This memory is so vivid I can smell the scent of greenery in the air from the nearby trees, the sun is creating rainbows of colours as it reflects off objects around me, and I'm somehow extremely aware of my surroundings. As an adult, I've spoken to my mother and father about this extremely vivid memory and have come to realise this was the day my father came home from prison. This was the day I became aware that the man we had visited in prison was my father.

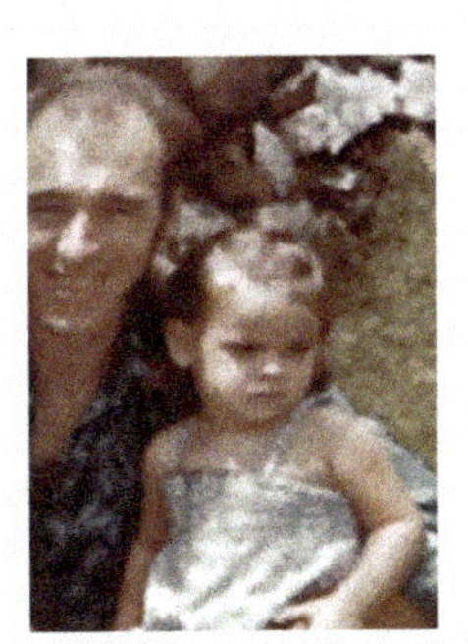

Meeting my dad

Dad was always in trouble when he was young, having had several scrapes with the law; hanging around with questionable characters often got him into trouble. Dad didn't seem to have the best upbringing. He told stories of being given three bullets and if he didn't come back with three dead rabbits to eat he would be beaten with a piece of 4x2 wood. He also spoke about truancy, throwing tomatoes at trains and all the general mischief he used to get up to. His mother died when he was in his late teens from what I suspect may have been a uterine cancer caused by invasive placental tissue (choriocarcinoma). This loss seemed to have a profound effect on him.

Dad used to reflect on how she died from a pregnancy gone wrong and that she just should have stopped having children. His mother had several different partners and he only had one full sibling to my knowledge. He idolised his mother but seemed to have a conflicted attachment to her, with anger directed at her, relating to all her partners and pregnancies.

Mum was in her late teens when she met Dad. According to Mum, she had already suffered horribly, having never known a healthy relationship in her young life. To me, it always seemed that if evil had a face, it would be that of her father. Thankfully, Mum made sure I spent very little time with him, but it was enough for me to feel how evil he truly was for myself. Mum was naive, damaged and vulnerable, and Dad, by all accounts, was charismatic and capable. He was so confident in his own capabilities that he could convince you of anything.

They were living together in regional Victoria, running a bantam chicken farm (according to Dad) when one of the questionable characters he spent time with became his partner in crime in what Dad described as a three-state car-stealing racket. Dad was apprehended in Tasmania trying to sell one of many of his stolen vehicles. My understanding is that he spent some time in Hobart's Risdon Prison and was then extradited to Victoria where he was able to get out on remand. While Dad was out on remand, Mum fell pregnant with me. Dad was eventually extradited to Queensland to face similar charges and spent time in Brisbane's notorious Boggo Road Gaol. While we did visit Dad when he was in prison, Mum said that I didn't really like him. Apparently, I was only two when Dad was released from prison. I only knew this man from visiting the prison with Mum. Suddenly, I was expected to accept him as my father and be happy for him to move in and live with us. As a two-year-old, who was very attached to my then single mother, I wasn't too keen on accepting this new person into our family. At the time, my father was also a very difficult man who, when challenged, would get physically aggressive. By all accounts, I took a disliking to how he treated

Mum. Also, his difficulty integrating back into society after more than two years in some tough prisons made it challenging for us to develop a relationship.

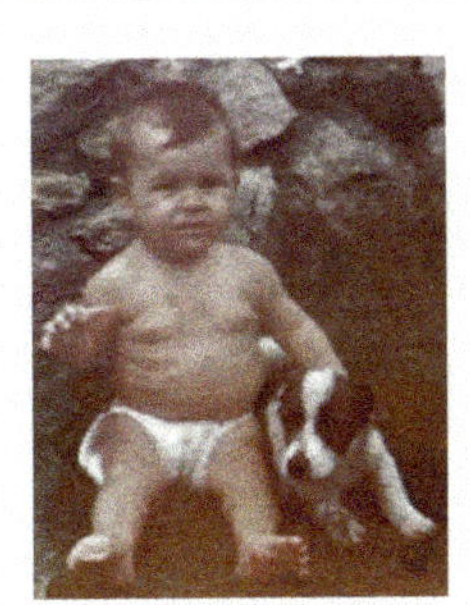
Where my love of dogs started

I can't imagine what this time was like for my mother. She was a single parent in the 1970s taking care of her little family both financially and physically. Mum had to work at a pub to make ends meet, getting a close friend, Sally, to care for me while she was at work. In her time off, we would travel by bus to the prison to visit Dad. My mother told me she had suffered terribly when she was young, and now she was a single parent having to earn money and visit her partner in prison.

The early days with Dad back at home were tumultuous, but Mum and Dad remained together, and we remained a family unit. I was four years old when they finally got married. I can remember the day vividly. Dad was in a typical 1970s purple suit with flared pants and sideburns. Mum was dressed in the most elegant, straight, white gown with exposed arms and a full length, hooded lace veil with sleeves and a train that extended beyond the bottom of her dress around a metre behind her on the floor. I was a flower girl, dressed in a long, straight, pink dress with a small section of rouching across the chest. I distinctly remember Mum standing me on what I think was a chest freezer to straighten my dress and check I was all ready for the ceremony. I remember looking up

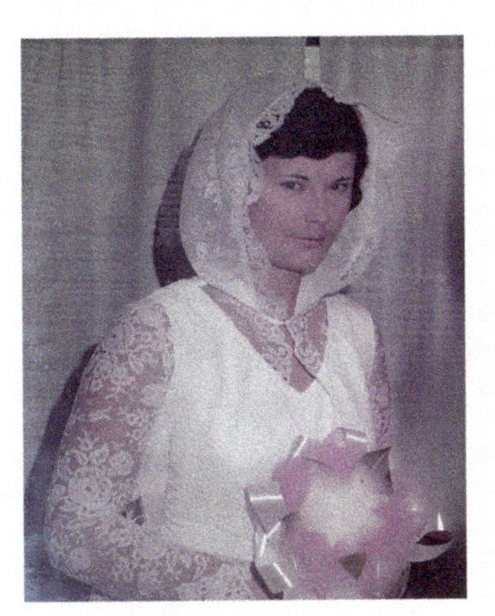
My beautiful Mum on her wedding day

at her face and thinking how absolutely stunning she looked in that long, flowing, hooded lace veil.

I always felt privileged to have been present that day and to have witnessed my mother and father's marriage with eyes old enough to remember. However, it wasn't the typical fairy tale the pictures seemed to depict. Dad was known for having a roving eye and there were many times in my childhood when I remember witnessing this for myself. One of the people at the wedding party was, according to Mum, a focus for one of these episodes of infidelity and, again, I can't imagine what this was like for my mother. In addition, there was always the threat of physical violence should Mum challenge his behaviour.

The 1970s was a very different time. When I was young, children were often left to their own devices to play and this was certainly a frequent occurrence in my upbringing, often leading to misadventure. I was just four years old when I heard the whistle of the kettle and ran, dressed only in my underwear and a white singlet, giggling in excitement as I tried to be the quickest to turn it off. I stepped up onto a stool and reached my little arms out towards the kettle and saw Mum out the corner of my eye, hurtling towards me, trying to catch me before I got to it. I was still giggling and trying to beat her to it when I accidentally pulled the kettle over, spilling boiling water all over the right side of my chest. I distinctly remember Mum peeling the singlet off as I screamed and cried, then grabbing the butter, cotton wool and a brown paper bag to dress the burn before bundling me up and taking me to the doctor. The smell of the butter and my burnt flesh will always stay with me. I still bear the scar of that burn on my right breast.

I believe I was only five years old when the next misadventure occurred in the absence of parental supervision. I was playing with a neighbourhood friend in my house when she decided it would be a good idea to put some bobby pins into the electrical socket.

I remember her saying, "Now you hold this and I'll turn it on."

As I dutifully held the bobby pin in the electrical socket, she turned on the switch. A burning pain shot up the index and middle fingers of my right hand, rapidly travelling up to my shoulder and into my chest. I was flung backwards across to the other side of the room where my back slammed hard against the wall. I saw Mum racing in to check on me as I was propped up against the wall, dazed and confused. She seemed relatively calm but everything in the minutes after being electrocuted was a haze. Mum observed me for the afternoon, keeping a close eye on me, but I don't remember being taken to the doctor. That just seemed to be how you did things in those days.

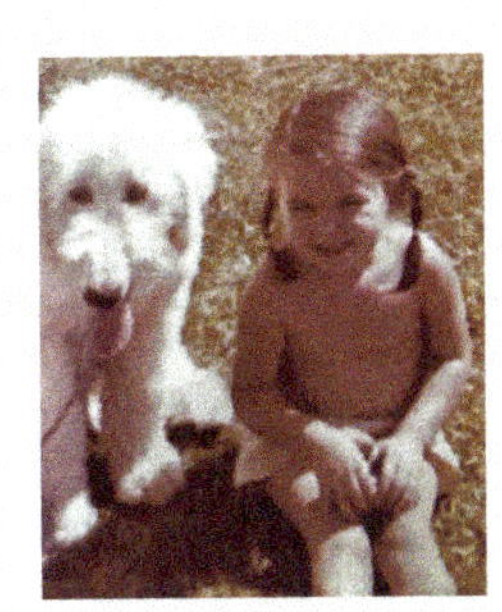

With one of Mum's show dogs

The ongoing struggle to support the family after Dad was released from prison had taken its toll. People weren't very understanding of Dad's prison time; he was essentially unemployable. As a result, I was always sworn to secrecy about family matters. They were private and should never be discussed outside the home! I just did what I was told at the time but I now understand this as a feature of coercive control. After a failed business venture in Queensland, Dad decided it was time to move on and try to make a go of it elsewhere. They would move back to Tasmania to be near Dad's brother who was a resourceful man with the same detailed knowledge of car mechanics and panel beating as Dad. At this stage of life, Mum really didn't have much of a voice and I don't recall her ever opposing what Dad decided to do. I think she learnt if you oppose him, there would be consequences and she had experienced what it was like to fend for herself.

What I didn't understand at the time is that Dad wanted to do this alone, just the two of them. At age six, I was dropped off at Mum's friend Sally's house while my parents left for Tasmania to make a new start. I remember being extremely upset and not having any clue as to when or even if they would ever return. I felt abandoned, unwanted, unloved and of no use to anyone. Sally was a beautiful woman and was always very kind. It didn't stop the yearning to have our little family back together, however dysfunctional that might be.

Six months after I was left at Sally's house, I developed a severe case of the mumps. I remember Mum calling to talk to me while I was sick. I was so grateful to hear her voice. It was nearly my seventh birthday and I missed her so much I ached on the inside. I missed Dad as well, but I was a sick six-year-old yearning for the care, love and support of her mother.

Mum would say things to me on the phone like, "Don't worry – I *will* come back for you."

This just made me think: *Does that mean there's a chance she* won't *come back?* I was lying in bed with a very swollen face, feeling extremely unwell on my seventh birthday, when I heard a knock at the door and through that door came the beaming, smiling face of my beautiful mother. She came to wish me a happy birthday and brought with her a bright blue dressing gown as a gift. Mum spent some time with me that day, but I was very unwell so I don't remember much. I know I cried in her arms, begging her to take me with her when she left, and she promised me that she'd be back.

After she left, I stared at the beautiful blue dressing gown on the back of the door to the bedroom I was sleeping in at Sally's house. Somehow, I just knew she'd be back soon and we'd be a family again. As I recall, it was a few months before I was put on a plane to Tasmania, being cared for by the air hostesses, to join Mum and Dad. Some other people I didn't know greeted me at the airport and I stayed at their house for another couple of months before being able to properly join them, initially in a caravan park and then in a house in a tiny town outside of Launceston.

This tiny little home had at least three bedrooms, a cosy little fireplace, a garage underneath and a lovely little backyard. It almost felt too good to be true. We were a normal suburban family living in the typical suburban family home. I was so relieved to be together as a family again and to feel normal. I was still seven years old when we moved into this house. Mum kept her promise. It must have been so difficult for my father to reintegrate into society after being in prison for so long. He had finally been able to bring his family together and find a way to financially support us to be in the same place. I was, of course, still sworn to secrecy about his time in prison, never being allowed to discuss it with him or anyone else. I have some beautiful memories of this little home; I remember it being the first time I felt relaxed and able to just be a child. There was still disharmony between Mum and Dad with frequent fighting that occasionally led to a physical altercation. He didn't frequently hit me, but he seemed to have a particular disdain towards me, and when he did hit me, it was very painful and often felt out of proportion to the degree of wrongdoing.

I remember several times scurrying into my bedroom after I'd done something I knew was wrong, expecting to get hit by my father with either the belt or the old-fashioned rope-like jug cord. I'd hear Dad's footsteps clumping hard on the floor as he came down the hall, huffing and mumbling angrily under his breath. If he was holding the belt, it was across his two hands folded over, flicking and making that awful cracking noise the belt would make as the two sides snapped onto each other, reminiscent of the noise it makes as it snaps onto your flesh. The sound of the snapping belt would make me shiver, replicating the feeling of it hitting my skin even if it wasn't in sight. Whenever I heard this noise coming, I'd crawl under the bed and get as far up against the wall as I possibly could in the hope he wouldn't be able to get to me, though of course that never worked. He would just drag me out by one foot then hit me with the belt. The jug cord was usually used if it was in reach. That thing drove fear into my heart; I would run as soon as he reached for it. Again, there was no chance of outrunning him – he always caught up with me.

One day my parents were play fighting when Dad picked up the jug cord he used for discipline and hit Mum with it. As Dad lunged forward, laughing and chasing Mum, he flicked the jug cord towards her, hitting Mum on the fleshy part of her upper thigh as she ran away. It took her breath away. She stopped and sat on the floor, catching her breath and holding her leg with tears streaming down her face. In this moment you could see the appreciation of the pain I must have suffered each time he hit me with that jug cord. In one of the first times I can remember Mum asserting herself and sticking up for me, she made him promise never to use the jug cord for discipline again. Though the belt still did the rounds, I was never hit with the jug cord again.

It wasn't too long after the jug cord incident that I witnessed Dad hit Mum for the last time. As was often the case, it started with a play fight but ended with Dad pushing Mum against the walls, yelling at her and slapping her. I don't recall him hitting her with a closed fist, but I do know from talking to Mum this frequently happened in the early days of their relationship. I had escaped to my room to stay well out of the way. I knew from experience it was a good idea to be as far away as possible when Mum and Dad were fighting like this. When everything was quiet and I felt like it was safe to come out of my room again, I ventured into the kitchen. There, at the top of the stairs to the garage, stood Mum with her bags packed, ready to leave.

"I've had enough and I'm never coming back," she sobbed.

He looked shocked and begged, "Please don't go Soosie – it was an accident."

He always minimised his behaviour. I remember sobbing and begging Mum not to go, clinging tightly to her leg. I didn't want to be separated from her again. Dad was also begging her not to go. She was adamant she would leave and never return if he ever laid a hand on her again. He promised it would never happen again and managed to convince her to stay. To his credit, he never physically struck Mum again. He threw plates and Coke bottles, and broke things, but never hit her again. It was a lesson in power and control. I logged in my brain how

Mum had been able to find the strength to stand up to Dad in that moment. I wasn't so brave and I wouldn't be so lucky, either!

I've spoken to Mum several times as an adult about this day, mostly to confirm I remembered it correctly. She reflected how surprised she was that standing up to Dad worked. She was so proud of herself for having the courage to do this despite the obvious risk of severe consequences. Her physical suffering at his hands may have ended but his coercive control would continue throughout their relationship. Power and fear had become weapons, and Dad would just find new ways to wield them. Mum was doing what she knew. This behaviour was nothing new to her. She had very little control and very rarely had a say in anything we did. Mum once told me she didn't even have an inner voice until she was 33 years old. It was then that she started her own journey of rebuilding and recovery, which was such an inspiration to me growing up. I believe people who are victimised as children are often drawn to abusive personalities in adulthood and I think this was true for Mum. While Dad wasn't evil by any means, by his own admission, his treatment of Mum during their relationship was "unforgiveable".

Unfortunately, it was around this time that Dad's friend, Dwayne, and his family drifted back into our lives. I always found him rather unsavoury, stout and creepy with his thick beard and dark sense of humour. Dad always flew close to the edge when it came to the law and his reassociation with Dwayne meant that he would come ever closer. I was about eight when Dad did something to upset him, and it didn't seem to take much to upset Dwayne. We were quietly going about our day in this lovely little house, I was inside playing and Mum and Dad were doing something off in the lounge room, when there was a knock at the door. I saw two grown men with sawn-off shotguns in their hands and black balaclavas over their heads. They were unrecognisable, very angry and wanted to see Dad.

Mum ushered me down the stairs and out the garage to the street front while Dad faced these two armed gunmen alone. I remember being very frightened and Mum holding me extremely tight, with her hands covering my ears while we waited to hear the gunshots and to see if Dad made it out alive. After several minutes we could hear laughter coming from upstairs, which was extremely confusing given the circumstances. Mum went upstairs to investigate and then called me in, saying everything was okay now. As I entered the lounge room, I could see Dwayne and another friend of Dad's sitting on either side of him, each with a cup of tea in hand, with the shotguns leaning up against the chair and the balaclavas on the bench. My eight-year-old brain had no way to make sense of this situation as I heard all three of them joking and laughing. Until his dying day, Dad would insist that this was just a joke done in poor taste by two mates.

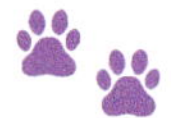

While we lived in this house I attended a lovely little rural school. There were animals all around, old-fashioned classrooms with wooden desks and ink wells, and pretend inspections of your fingernails and skirt length – all of which gave us a glimpse into what it was like for kids in the "olden days". I had friends and loved seeing the animals, so it was a happy time for me, but things were still difficult at home. When Dad was annoyed with me, he would frequently either hit me over the head or kick me up the backside. He seemed to get some joy out of watching me tuck my bum in and duck my head as I walked past. One day I was supposed to be at school participating in the cross country, but I convinced Mum to let me stay home. I don't remember what triggered Dad. It seemed like he was irritated by my apathy towards cross country and generally just annoyed at having me home. I don't think I was aware how annoyed he was because I walked past him and forgot to duck my head or tuck my bum in. He had filthy, brown, reinforced work boots, covered in paint and mud, on at the time and he kicked me hard as I strolled by. This time it hit my vulva, not my backside.

Winded, I held my hand over my bottom so he couldn't do it again and hobbled to my bedroom as fast as I could, crying and trying to get my breath back. His favourite words for me were "idiot" or "stupid" and later in life "subordinate". His choice this time was idiot.

I could hear him taunting, "You idiot! You should have moved faster" as I ran to my bedroom, slamming the door behind me. I took this as a reference to avoiding the cross-country race. Sobbing in my bedroom, I could feel something warm and wet in my pants. I thought I wet myself. I waited until the coast was clear and gingerly hobbled to the bathroom, careful to avoid running into Dad. When I got to the toilet, I saw blood.

While this scared me, I was too frightened to tell Dad, and Mum was out so I couldn't tell her. I folded up some toilet paper and put it in my pants hobbling back to my bedroom, shutting the door behind me. When she came home, I told Mum what happened, and with love and care she took a look. There was nothing to see, the bleeding had stopped. She told Dad he wasn't allowed to kick me up the backside anymore. *In future*, I reasoned, *I need to be smarter! Dad's right. What an idiot not to tuck my backside in and protect myself!* This was the beginning of the little voice in my head that told me how stupid I was.

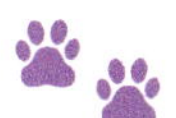

Not long after moving into this house, we purchased a Great Dane puppy. I believe Dad wanted the Great Dane primarily for protection given the quality of some of the people he spent time with and the recent incident of Dwayne and the guns. Our dog, Grace, was very well trained and defended the house and the family. I recall one night Dad cooked something in fat in the oven and forgot about it, leaving the oven on long after we'd gone to bed. Grace came to my bed in the middle of the night and licked my face. I opened my eyes to see Grace's face and was quickly overcome by thick, black smoke. I started to cough, my eyes stinging as I raced to Mum and Dad's bedroom. They were already getting out of bed; Grace was well ahead of me.

The kitchen was on fire! As the flames spread up the kitchen curtains, I will never forget watching Dad trying to put them out in his underwear with nothing but a bucket of water. I have no idea how he managed to do it but he extinguished the flames, the fire unable to spread beyond the kitchen. This was a rental property and the entire kitchen had to be gutted and redone. However, Dad, being the incredible handyman he was, somehow managed to make this happen without too great an impact on our finances. This was one of the most amazing things about my father. He was an incredibly difficult man, but he could turn his hand to just about anything. He was creative, he could solve just about any problem you put in front of him. He had an innate ability to visualise something in its finished state before he even began work on it. This is a gift my father passed down to me and one I'm very grateful for.

While Grace was an incredible watchdog and protector, she could also be incredibly destructive. One night we went out to the Speedway with Dwayne and his family, who also had a Great Dane. We left them locked up in the garage with food, water and some toys. I don't think we thought for a second there would be any problem. We were quite sure the Great Danes would keep the house safe. What we probably failed to appreciate is the house might have needed protecting from the Great Danes! When we arrived home, we came in through the garage to find no dogs and a door that had been chewed to pieces. We followed the debris up the stairs and into the kitchen, turning into the lounge room to find everything, and I mean everything, upturned or chewed. We proceeded into the bedrooms one

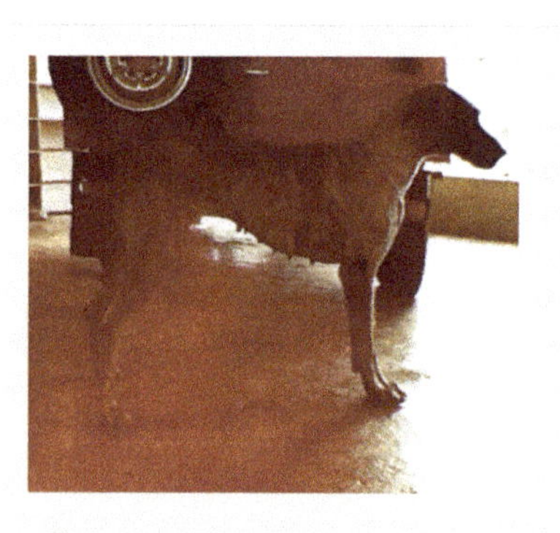

Beautiful Grace in the garage

by one only to find each mattress overturned, clothes and other items strewn all over the floor, and Mum's favourite slippers in tiny little pieces spread over each bedroom. The dogs were wagging their tails, happy to see us and proud of the mess they made. Needless to say, we never left them alone in the house again. This dog was my first great animal love. I've had an affinity for dogs and Great Danes ever since. Sadly, when we moved out of this house, we moved into a caravan out the back of a factory so we couldn't take her with us. Everything was disposable when it came to Dad and animals were no different. He found a home on a property somewhere nearby and we never saw Grace again, which broke my heart. I still think about Grace from time to time and how hard that transition must have been for her.

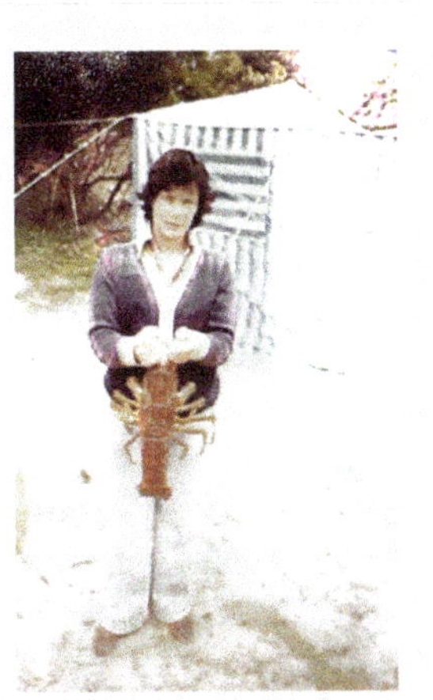

Mum holding the huge crayfish Dad caught

I'm not sure why we moved into a caravan out the back of a factory, but I believe it was because Dad got work there and we needed to be closer to his job. Dad was a gun enthusiast, so we always had weapons in the house. He was also an avid hunter, shooting, catching or trapping a lot of what we ate. I think I've had kangaroo and rabbit cooked in every way possible. On the upside, this often meant we had fresh seafood, which I absolutely loved and still do.

I was also taught from a very young age how to store, load and fire a gun accurately. Dad always told me if you feel threatened you shoot first and ask questions later. I guess for him this made sense; he was always on the wrong side of someone and always looking over his shoulder. The living conditions in this little caravan weren't great. It was cramped with no room and no privacy. Mum got a new dog at the other end of the extreme, a Chihuahua named Honey for her honey-coloured coat. I had a new friend; someone to play with who wanted to play

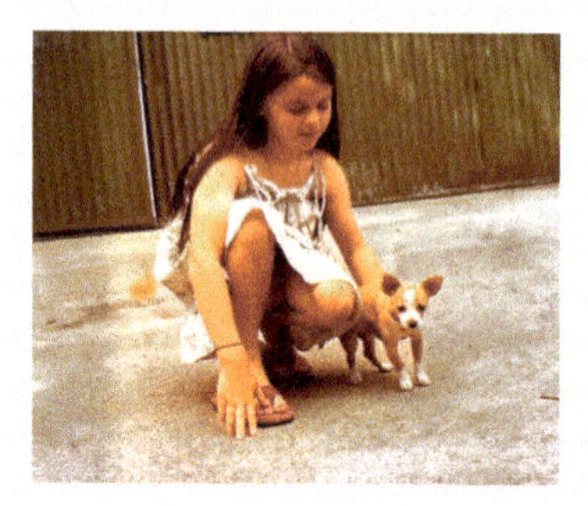
With Honey outside the factory

with me. I remember being so lonely as a child and the dogs were always great company. I could tell them anything and they never seemed to get angry at me. I genuinely felt loved by animals. I always understood them better than I understood people.

I remember this as an unstable time in our lives. Unfortunately, there was usually someone unhappy with Dad because the quality of his work wasn't what they expected or because the deal went wrong and they felt ripped off in some way. He always seemed to be running from someone or something. We always seemed to be extremely poor and struggled to make ends meet from week to week. Mum used to talk about times when she only had flour, milk and jam in the house and we'd live off scones for the week until Dad got some money. Most of Dad's work was doing up cars or boats or other things he could buy at a low price and, with little effort, sell at a higher price. He called himself a wheeler dealer and took pride in being able to turn something ordinary into something better and make money in the process.

While we were in this little caravan, I started to push the boundaries of behaviour. I remember one day several of Dad's friends were over, talking about cars as they usually did, when one of them really annoyed me with his disrespectful tone. I turned around and said loudly, "You're a prick!"

I'd only heard someone say this word for the first time a few days earlier and I knew it was nasty but had no real idea of its meaning. I was eight; it could have meant anything for all I knew. Dad overheard this and, when I saw him coming, I knew I was in trouble. I scurried away and we danced around the old beat-up car in the driveway until he finally caught me by the hair.

He dragged me away, spitting and hissing, "I'll teach you."

His rage was evident on his face. I had embarrassed him. I had no clue what was coming next but it was a new, special kind of torture I would learn to avoid at all costs. Still pulling my hair, he dragged me to the filthy little sink in the toilet of this factory shed, held my head over the tap and turned it on. I pulled away as much as I could but his grip on my hair just tightened with every pull. *Is he going to drown me?* Fearing what would come next, I continued to struggle against the restraint. Then he took the filthy, foamy cake of soap from the sink and shoved it deep in my mouth. I gagged as he rubbed it around, ensuring the soap lathered up in my mouth.

"Don't you ever say that word again!" he said as he walked away, leaving me with the cake of soap oozing out of my mouth, the water still running. As Dad returned to his mates, I could hear them laughing and joking around. I rinsed my mouth out but it just kept foaming with soap. It took several minutes to stop gagging and to clear my mouth of the suds. This punishment was very effective and would be for several years to come. To this day I feel the discomfort in the back of my throat when I tell this story and I still don't swear very much because of the trauma associated with having my mouth washed out with soap.

We were still living in the caravan when Mum went on a short trip away. Honey and I were left with Dad to take care of us and he did a pretty good job. Towards the end of her time away, we went to a house party. At this party, I believe I saw with my own eyes the infidelity Mum had complained of for so many years. Dad recurrently gaslit Mum about this infidelity, telling her it was all in her head and she was just jealous. At this party, a woman was falling all over Dad, constantly touching and caressing his legs, kissing his cheek, coming on to him and insisting on spending time with him alone.

As a young girl, I found this gross! This lady came in the car with us to the caravan where Dad dropped me off to "take her home". It was several hours before he returned. I stayed up, worried about him since he had been gone for so long. I was so frightened I checked the handgun and ammunition, so I knew where it all was if someone came to the van.

This was well before mobile phones and there was no public phone anywhere near this industrial estate. There was no way to contact him to check and see if he was okay. I just had to wait for him to get home. When he got home I was awake and angry, worried something had happened to him and frightened for my own safety. It felt obvious, even to an eight-year-old, he had been unfaithful to Mum in some way that night. I knew it wasn't the first time, and I knew it wasn't going to be the last, but this time I knew I was going to tell Mum when she got home from her trip. It was a hard conversation but I think she had come to expect this kind of behaviour from him.

This and Dad's response to Mum's questions shattered whatever respect I had for him. I couldn't understand how he could treat Mum so badly. I listened intently as he made excuses and blamed her for overreacting to what was clearly an innocent attempt to help someone get home safely when they were inebriated. I watched him lie with great confidence about the details of the party and his interactions with this lady, knowing full well what the truth was. I watched him get angry with her and somehow convince her this was her problem. In the end she was apologising to him for questioning his fidelity. Without knowing it, that day I learnt what narcissism is. I also learnt that speaking up would only hurt Mum.

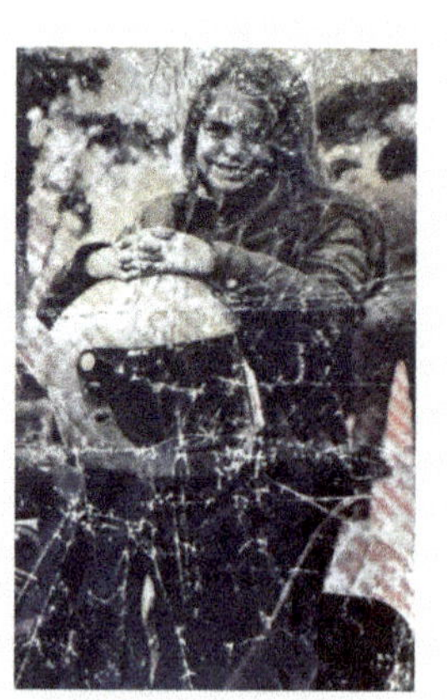

My five minutes of fame - sitting on top of my kart with my helmet

While Mum and Dad were often in conflict, they also did a lot of fun things together. Dad was always interested in fast cars and racing was something he always enjoyed. Most of our spare money went into Dad's latest and greatest adventure. Go-kart racing was one of his passions. He had a go-kart, before we knew it Mum had one, and then I showed interest so I got one too. Dad was always disappointed in my racing; I just didn't have the drive to win. I was too careful. At age eight, I was featured in a local paper as the youngest female go-kart racer in Tasmania.

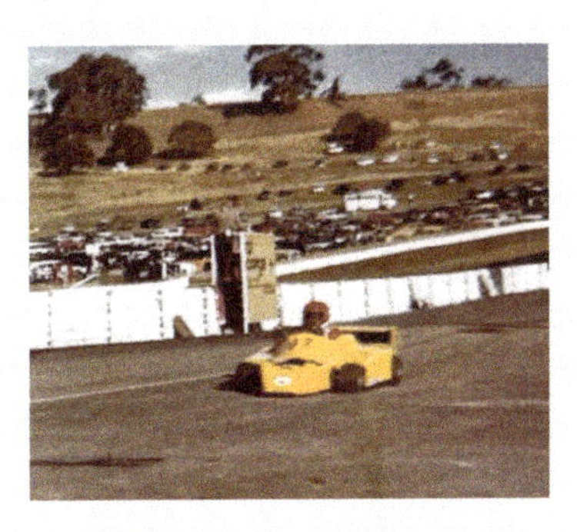

Dad in his superkart

I never even won a race but this five minutes of fame made Dad look good, so for me it was about trying to make him proud. Dad made the engines himself and made sure they were the fastest in the field. When I wasn't racing, I was helping out in the pits, lap scoring or in the commentator's box. We always had an engine part in the oven drying out, much to Mum's annoyance. Mum won many of the women's races and Dad won in his divisions. Mum's trophy was bigger than Dad's, which was a sore point we teased him about whenever we knew we could get away with it. I spent a lot of time when I was young showing interest in whatever Dad was interested in so I could win his approval. I don't think I ever did but I tried for many years, even into adulthood, in the hope that one day he would be proud of me.

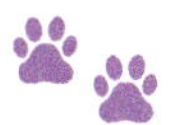

I was nine or 10 years old when Mum and Dad bought their first house. It was a little cottage in a suburb of Launceston. Dad set about renovating it while we lived in one section. It always fascinated me watching Dad at work. He was truly talented with his hands and could make just about anything come to life from a simple idea. My room was the former lounge and the last one to be renovated. The chimney was still open and the room was freezing cold, a throwback to the history of this little cottage. I started going to a little primary school nearby.

This was to be the 11th primary school I attended and the last. Dad did a great job of the renovations, turning the house into a cosy little cottage we called home. One of the common features of my upbringing was being left at home alone. As I got older, this became more frequent; I was always curious as to why I couldn't go with my parents when they went out. Sometimes I would sneak into the car to force the issue but I'd inevitably get caught and end up in trouble with Dad so it was never worth it. When they were at home, I was reminded "children should be seen and not heard", as the saying goes.

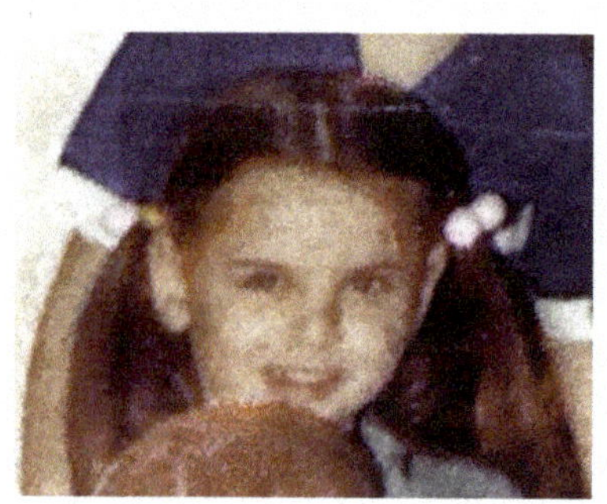

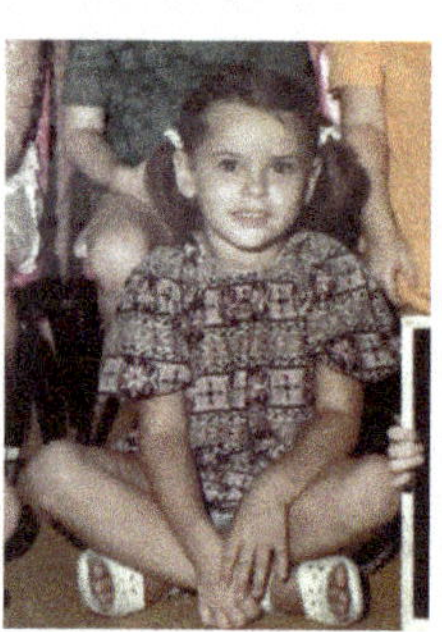

Class photos at two of the 11 primary schools I attended

Close to my 11th birthday, I told Mum I wanted to earn some money so I could save up for an upcoming trip away. With Mum's blessing, I approached a little garage near our home and asked if I could help clean by sweeping the floor to earn a little bit of pocket money. The owner agreed and I started working there. I also earned extra money picking wild raspberries, blackberries and mulberries, and selling them to neighbours. It was around this time that, despite my mother's best efforts to protect me, I would learn how vulnerable young girls are around adult males.

The owner of this little garage would allow me to sweep his floors for 50 cents every Saturday. As a very young girl, my perception is that this man was very tall. He had dark hair, was slightly overweight and probably in his early 30s. He had been fun, jovial and kind ever since I'd known him. I knew all about stranger danger, but he was the father of one of my old school friends, so I had no reason to be afraid of this man or to think that he would do me harm. I was sweeping the floor as I always did every Saturday. I was dressed in a long-sleeve shirt and warm, loose fitting, fleecy lined track pants. He had earlier made an innocent comment about how my track pants must be very warm to which I replied, "Yes, they are." He made comments before about how pretty I was. As a well-developed 11-year-old, I frequently heard such comments, so I thought nothing of them.

I had almost finished my work, and was just about to bend down to scoop the dust into the dustpan, when this man came up behind me very quickly, wrapping his long arms around my waist and putting his filthy, greasy hands down the front of my pants, saying, "Is it warm enough for me in there?" I pulled away instantly but said nothing. I could smell the mechanics grease combined with dust and paint, and sensed him staring at me, watching my every move. There was a tension in the air that I desperately wanted to escape from, but I had to finish my job!

Dad indoctrinated in me a strong work ethic. One of his favourite sayings was, "If a job's worth doing, it's worth doing properly." I finished picking up the dust I had swept up as quickly as I could, he handed me my 50 cents, and I ran home. It's so interesting to me as an adult that I stayed and finished the job I had been paid for despite what this man had just done. In hindsight, I had been conditioned to do as I was told or suffer the consequences. Children were to be seen and not heard and, in my world, male adults had ultimate power. I was frightened and I feel lucky now that it didn't escalate further and I was able to get away. It just goes to show you don't know how you're going to react to something until it happens to you, and you might not react the way you think you're going to.

I distinctly remember a loud voice in my head, repeating all the way home: *If I was fat and ugly, this would never have happened to me.* Food would become my security blanket, and gaining weight my safety buffer, from unwanted attention. This would begin a lifelong battle with my weight, which is ongoing to this day. I immediately told Mum about what had happened and she advised me never to go there again. I know she told Dad but I'm unaware of the outcome for the man. I just know I had to pass this man every day going to and from school, but he never once even looked in my direction again. I'm quite sure Dad threatened him in some way. For once, I was grateful for his aggressive responses. I always felt guilty, knowing what kind of man this person was, that I didn't disclose to someone else because I was pretty sure if he was happy to do this to me, he was probably doing it to others.

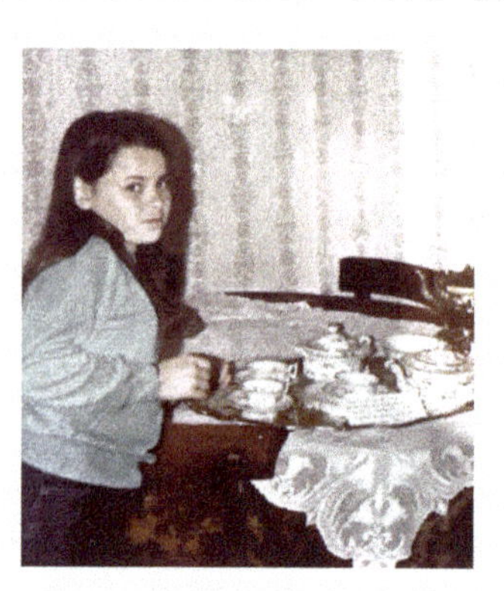

Around age 10-11

As a young, vulnerable girl with working parents who were often absent, I was a sitting duck for this kind of exploitation. Even at school, I didn't feel safe. In one of the many primary schools I attended as a child, it was commonplace for boys to chase girls, hold them down and finger them. The girls seemed to be aware that this was happening and the boys would taunt them throughout the day. I was aware that it usually happened out of sight of teachers, and the most common place was on a bench in the dark passageway to the girls' toilets. I did my best to stay away from the girls' toilets during the day and this would become a habit that extended into adulthood. Public toilets were a place to avoid if you were alone. I got away with it by asking to use the toilet during class, whenever I absolutely had to go, but understandably the teachers would often get upset if you asked to go to the toilet just after the break. Sadly, the day came that I just had to go at recess – I was busting! I waited until I knew there was no-one in that passageway and ran as quickly as I could into the toilets.

Unfortunately, as I was exiting the toilet, the boys were waiting for me. There were four of them and they were much bigger and stronger than me. I knew what was about to happen and I think that made it worse. I still tried to run around them, smiling and laughing nervously in an attempt to defuse the situation, the best my young brain could come up with at the time. I remember the sense of powerlessness I felt as I was fighting and screaming for them to stop while being held down by these much stronger boys for what seemed like an eternity but in reality was probably less than a minute. I never told anyone. I didn't tell any teachers. I didn't even tell Mum. I reasoned: *You should have been smarter. You know those boys are bad news.*

By then I was well and truly convinced that anything that happened to me was my fault. I never thought of this as a sexual assault. It was just so common. Such inappropriate touching had happened to many other girls I knew in one way or another, a sad reflection of the society we live in. Thankfully, this would be my last experience like this with these boys, as I never again dared to go to the toilet during break time. I always went during class time, regardless of how much it annoyed the teacher. Public toilets have been a problem for me ever since, they just don't feel safe.

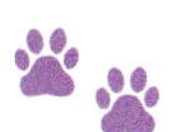

It was always a bit difficult to know where I stood with Mum when I was a child. While I always knew she loved me, some days she could be quite unpredictable with her emotions, which I put down to the strained relationship with Dad. She would often want me to be affectionate towards adults whether I liked them or not, expressing she felt it was impolite not to give a hug or kiss hello or goodbye. I often found this intrusive. Mum would also get upset if you didn't show her affection. One day, after a loud and ugly, typical rebellious teenage argument with her, in which I was admittedly very rude, I was sitting drawing when Mum approached and asked me for a kiss, to make up. When I declined and made a snide remark, she slapped me hard in the face, recounting how badly I'd treated her earlier as she marched me off to my room. At the time, I didn't understand Mum's need for validation and affection, nor did I understand the extent of her own trauma. I was stunned at the unfairness of this slap, burying myself in music to cope. She always apologised, which made her very different to Dad, but I learnt to be cautious of her mood. Even when she was in a good mood, she would sometimes play games that got me into trouble.

One of her favourite games to play was to pull faces behind Dad's back to get me to laugh. It was harmless and I believe Mum was just trying to lighten the mood a little, but then Dad would get mildly annoyed, I'd get yelled at, and she would look at me and laugh quietly. One day, this innocent little game got serious. Dad was in a particularly bad mood and Mum made me laugh as she usually did. But this time, seemingly out of nowhere, Dad slammed both hands on the table, lifting the dishes an inch off their position, and yelled at me, "Go to bed!"

I scurried off to bed without dinner that night and Dad refused to let me out or to relent, despite Mum explaining this was an innocent game. Mum did come in and apologise but I still got angry at her for getting me into trouble. While I was in the room by myself, I remember obsessively memorising my times tables while slapping my wrists. I found maths therapeutic as it was predictable – and predictability was something my life was sorely lacking. Slapping my wrists was an escape, a way to release the anger without getting into trouble. I'm grateful this didn't become a habit, but that night the physical pain of slapping myself gave me some relief from the internal pain I was feeling. This has given me a deep empathy for people who self-harm.

I was selling some of my raspberries to the local store one day when I saw my mum driving out of our street onto the road the shop was on. I wondered what she was doing. She yelled out to me, from the tiny Mini Cooper we owned at the time, "Have you seen Honey? She got out!"

"No."

She drove off as I joined the search for her. I wandered along the road and, just as Mum came back around the corner, I saw Honey. Mum opened the door of the car and yelled out to her angrily to come. I could see the oncoming car, but Mum was focused on Honey so she didn't see it. I yelled out to Mum but she didn't hear me. The car ran over Honey's tiny little Chihuahua frame. I couldn't do anything other than watch it happen. I screamed and cried at the same time, racing towards the car. Mum was inconsolable as she tried to rouse Honey but her body was limp. We went home unable to look at the carnage anymore. Mum asked Dad to go and pick her up because she just couldn't do it.

He grumbled, "I didn't want a bloody dog in the first place. You always get the animals, and I have to scrape them up out of the gutter!"

As I sobbed into my pillow, I could hear Electric Light Orchestra's *Telephone Line* blaring on the reel-to-reel (a large version of a tape recorder). I had lost my second pet love and confidant. I still can't listen to that song without tearing up. I always had an affinity for animals; they made me feel safe. You could tell them everything, they never told anyone else and they always seemed to love you no matter how bad a day you were having. Honey was gone and I knew it would be a long time before Dad would let us have another pet!

DADDY, DON'T HURT ME

I met you when I was just two, we didn't have the best start
But I still wonder how my cheeky little grin didn't melt you heart
I would look up to you every time I saw your face
Hoping to feel love only to be denied your embrace
I was only a child, I never meant any disrespect
I wondered why, in your eyes, I was so easy to reject
I thought the jug cord or the belt was bad enough
But kicking a child when they're down, that was pretty rough
I loved you then and still do to this day
But the bruises run deep, the pain I wasn't allowed to say
I remember your cold hard stare and that sense of dread
When you got angry with me and I used to hide under the bed
You were both a hero and the boogie man in my little eyes
But you were also my daddy, why didn't you hear my cries?
When I grew big and strong enough to fight back
That was the last time I would feel the sting of your smack
I'm an adult now, mother of two babies of my own
It makes me wonder: was your heart really made of stone?
How could you hurt your little girl so often at your own hand
This I have spent my whole life trying to understand
You can no longer hurt me, of this I'm now sure
But I'm not like you and my love for you will endure
Daddy, I forgive you for all the bad things you did to me
I didn't end up like you, that mere fact has set me free

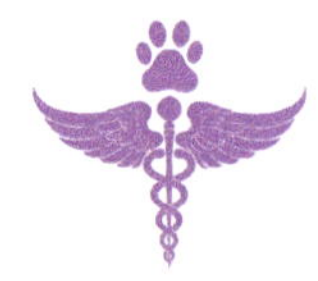

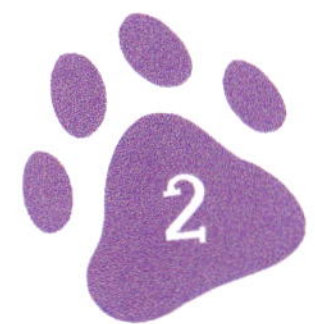

I was so excited to go to high school! I had a few friends going to the same school and I loved the idea of being part of a big school community. It wasn't the best school, but we couldn't afford those. As was usually the case, we didn't have any money to buy uniforms, good shoes, the right books or any other school-related equipment. Dad always had money to buy the next racing gadget or keep the kart or racing car going but we often had no money for food or other necessities. As we were preparing for me to start high school, I remember going to the op-shop to get my uniform and shoes. I didn't care that they were different at the time; I didn't understand the impact this would have on my socialisation at high school.

One day while shopping, I remember pointing out to Mum that she should buy herself some new underwear. It hadn't escaped my notice that Dad had everything he wanted and needed but Mum didn't even have underwear without holes in them. I tried to encourage her to buy herself some new underwear this day, but she wouldn't budge, stating she didn't need new underwear and we were here to buy things for my high school. This is one of the characteristics I remember Dad saying he loved about Mum. She had modest needs at best and she never made any demands. He used to tell a story of a day when he brought home thousands of dollars in cash and threw it on the bed proudly telling Mum, "You can have whatever you want. What do you want to buy?"

Dad said she couldn't think of a thing and refused to use the money for herself. Mum had learnt money was tight and while there were times Dad was flush with cash, those times were short-lived. She was frugal and sensibly planned for leaner times.

Mum always made the best out of what she had. One of the things I really admired about her was her ability to create something out of absolutely nothing. Often, we had nothing in the house to eat that would come close to creating a decent meal but somehow, there was always food on the table. This resourcefulness was something I took with me from my childhood that served me well. One day I was unloading the dryer and found a $50 note poking out of Dad's pants. I rushed it out to Mum, presenting it to her like it was a priceless gem.

"Shhh…don't tell your father," she instructed, and took me to the shop to buy lollies, cigarettes and some essentials. I felt like we won the lottery. Mum would later inform me she had no money for groceries that week and the $50 got us through the next two weeks, putting food on the table. Of course, $50 went a lot further in those days than it does now.

Despite my idealised view of high school as a fresh start, it was a nightmare for me both socially and academically. I was struggling to maintain focus, had only one good friend and suffered relentless bullying. There were so many reasons to bully me I'm not sure which one was most prominent. We were always poor, I never had a real uniform, I wasn't very bright in class, most of my clothes still had that op-shop feel and smell. While all the other kids had the latest gadget, shoes or toy, I only had my imagination to keep me company. The bullying, combined with the ongoing difficulty both financially and personally at home, led to recurrent truancy, poor academic performance and significant rebellion. Just like Dad had been, I was always in trouble! I'd already been offered cocaine and marijuana but had the common sense to decline.

Dad had a saying that echoed through my head: "You don't have to pour battery acid on yourself to know it's going to hurt."

I still use this saying today. Even at that age, I knew I didn't want whatever trouble drugs were going to bring me!

There was ongoing tension between myself and my father but I had begun fighting back. This tumultuous time came to a head when I was

13. I was now utterly convinced I was stupid. I had no hope of achieving anything at school and my social circle was ever shrinking. I was doing whatever I could to rebel – smoking, drinking, shoplifting (usually lollies) and anything else that might get the attention of my parents. Around this time, my mother started her own little business. Somewhere in the recesses of my mind, this made me think that as a young woman I could do anything. She was an inspiration to me and I thought maybe someday I could make her proud. It was obvious to my parents that things weren't going well for me at school when I was attacked on the school oval by one of the female school thugs and had to have X-rays of my jaw to make sure it wasn't broken. My father advised me I needed to learn how to fight back and stop just taking the beatings, but I was an absolute pacifist. I had no idea how to be aggressive, even in defence. My whole life I had learnt to be quiet, to shrink away when somebody (usually Dad) was aggressive. Otherwise, it got worse. This is all I knew how to do. The bullying continued and as it escalated so did my bad behaviour.

Around this time, I also began to develop an interest in boys, much to my mother and father's disgust. I was banned from having a boyfriend and wasn't allowed to wear makeup, so when my father found me one day, standing at a bus stop with makeup all over my face, dressed up to go out and meet my secret boyfriend, he was horrified. He got out of the car and grabbed me by the upper arm. "Come here, young lady," he said through gritted teeth as he dragged me into the car, absolutely humiliating me in front of my friends.

He took me home and forced me to scrub the makeup off my face, explaining how this made me look "easy" and it wasn't appropriate for his daughter. I was seething on the inside and found ways to bypass his rules, putting my makeup on and getting changed into the clothes I wanted to wear in the park around the corner, finding ways to meet up with my boyfriend and my other friends, even sometimes sneaking out the window at night.

I had a lovely boyfriend who was very respectful and kind. Not long after the bus stop incident, at one of our regular secret meetings, this boyfriend told me he loved me and as proof of that love he put a love bite on my neck. This was a very popular thing to do at the time and very common for girls my age. We were so innocent, and we never did anything other than kiss and canoodle. I loved how respectful and kind he was. Somehow my mum found out about this. When I got home from school that day, she told me how upset she was with me because I wasn't allowed to have a boyfriend, that she was going to tell Dad and that he'd be home to "deal with me" soon.

I understand why my mother was so careful about me not having boyfriends at this age, but I don't think she appreciated how disproportionate Dad's reaction would be. When Dad got home from work that afternoon, he took me out into our back shed and again yelled at me about how I was making myself look "easy" to boys and how they only had one thing on their mind. This time, I was arguing back. I was so sick of Dad telling me what to do, and as a teenager I was rebelling against these tight rules, particularly given how kind and caring my boyfriend was and how normal I knew this was for all the other girls in my grade.

Unfortunately, by fighting back I had enraged him. He hit me on every part of my arms and legs as hard as he possibly could. The blows just kept coming, one after the other. He was holding my arm so I couldn't get away. My skin was burning as it twisted under his ever-tightening grip. I was screaming and crying but yelling at him at the same time, angrily and defiantly trying to tell him, "I didn't do anything wrong."

His eyes were dark and empty, his lips pursed, teeth clenched and brow furrowed. He looked menacing. I was more frightened of him in that moment than I had ever been before. This was the face I imagined my mother had seen so many times before. He just kept hitting. At one point, we were next to the pool table we had in our back shed and, still holding my arm so I couldn't get away, he picked up the pool cue and swung it as hard as he possibly could, hitting me across my buttocks and breaking the pool cue in the process. This seemed to jolt him back into the present, I saw the fire in his eyes start to dwindle.

As he stopped hitting me, he said through gritted teeth, "You disgust me. Get out of my sight!"

He finally released his grip on my arm and I was able to escape him. Hurt and crying, I ran to my room and shut the door. I couldn't believe what had just happened. *Did my own father just beat me*? This wasn't like previous episodes of discipline that might have involved one or two hits. This went on for several minutes and left me bruised and sore from my shoulders to my knees. By the next day, the bruises were visible. I was so angry with Dad I wanted to get him in trouble so I showed everyone I could the finger marks, the bruises that extended from the top of my shoulder all the way down to my forearms, the bruises on my back and upper thighs, and even offered to show them the giant welt across my buttocks where he broke the pool cue over my tiny body. No-one did anything to protect me. I had lost faith in my mother as it felt like she had sent me in for this beating, knowing what Dad was like. I had no faith in the adults around me. *Why can no-one protect me?* I felt lost, alone and very angry! I started to hate my father and grew increasingly defiant as a result.

The year I turned 13 was one of the most difficult times in my life. I was hormonal, I thought I was stupid and would never make anything of myself and, because of my poor academic performance and behaviour at school, this was the rhetoric coming from the school as well. I was now regularly fighting back when my father called me "stupid" or "subordinate" (his favourite word for me now I was older). I was still being randomly smacked over the back of the head and, to a lesser extent, kicked up the backside when I passed by him. One day I needed some money to get hot chips to go with our dinner and Mum had asked me to go to Dad's work shed to pick up the money. I had a long, modest but tight little summer dress on I had worn several times before. Having just come from my good friend's house who just happened to be a boy. Dad took offence to me wearing this dress around my very platonic friend and started yelling again about how I dressed. I was absolutely sick of his crap by now and argued back with whatever disrespectful language I could think of, without swearing of course, telling him how out of touch and old he was. This led to my second beating.

After he started to hit me, I began to turn away but he kicked my back foot, tripping me so I would fall. He then started to hit and kick me while I lay on the ground. This time, there was no way I was going to cry or show weakness. That now familiar look of rage, dead eyes, gritted teeth and furrowed brow was staring back at me. In between his rage-filled hits and kicks, I sat up and looked him dead in the eyes and said, "Is that the best you've got?"

This stopped him in his tracks.

I got up to my feet staring him down and, as he backed away, I stepped forward and said defiantly through my own gritted teeth, "I thought so!"

Still maintaining direct eye contact, I backed away and then turned my back to him as if in disgust. I scurried away as soon as I was out of his line of sight. *I can't believe that worked!* I left there beaten and bruised but triumphant. I knew I caught him off guard and I could do it again if I needed to. Mum found out this had occurred. She asked me if I was okay and I reassured her. I felt confident that, just has Mum had done when I was younger, I had figured out how to handle him now and he never actually hit me again after that day. I had a chance to talk to him in my 20s about these beatings and he reluctantly apologised, adding he was glad he was so tough on me because it "made me strong".

It was also in this year that Dad decided it was time he explained "why your mother's like she is". They had been arguing about modesty (not coming out of the bathroom in a towel), now that I was beginning to develop. I saw this as pretty normal and really didn't know any different. However, one day after he'd had another argument with

Mum where she stormed off, he sat me down and told me all about the mistreatment Mum had suffered in her life and how this was the reason for her overprotective, erratic behaviour.

He then launched into a lecture about how "if you want to keep your man, you have to keep him satisfied". I think my eyes got tired as they recurrently rolled in the back of my head in utter disrespect for this vile description of how to "keep your man". This felt so wrong. Mum's story wasn't his to tell and the way he told it, along with his added "advice" about how to "keep your man", was so derogatory to Mum. However, it did help me to understand her a bit more and made me want to protect her. I was 15 years old before I told Mum about this conversation. She was devastated she wasn't given the chance to tell me her personal history herself and appalled at the description of Dad's lecture about "how to keep your man satisfied".

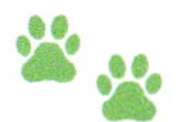

One night there was a very noisy concert going on nearby. Mum and I were watching *Grease*, the musical, on TV. Dad was out the back working when we heard a loud crash out the front. We went out to investigate, Dad discovered someone had thrown a Coke bottle through the windscreen of one of his many cars out the front of our house. There was glass everywhere and we assumed it was hooligans from the nearby concert. However, later that night when a car passed by out front, we were on alert. My mother did her usual peek through the curtains to see who it was and I peeked alongside her. We saw an old Holden sedan drive slowly past with a shotgun hanging out the passenger-side window, pointed towards the house. It suddenly seemed very chaotic. I had no idea what was happening, just that it seemed serious and very scary. Mum rushed out to alert Dad, ushering me into my room along the way. At the time, I was told that Dad had been involved in a dispute with someone he believed to be connected to the local drug trade. He had apparently reported this information anonymously as part of the first Operation Noah. This was a national police operation that allowed members of the public to anonymously call in tips to police about illegal drug use or trade.

It came as no surprise. In my mind, it seemed like the inevitable consequence of Dad's willingness to involve himself in situations that carried such risk. Mum put me under the bed in the back room of the house, barricaded the door and gave instructions to wait until she personally came back. I heard them debating what to do. Mum called the police and Dad went out in the Mini Cooper with a crowbar, seemingly intent on chasing the car away, leaving us in the house to fend for ourselves. I was so frightened, and it seemed like an eternity before Mum came back. When the police arrived they found the car abandoned at the back of our property. It was a long night, the police kept driving by and I don't think anyone slept. At some point, I was told the individual was later apprehended in relation to a separate matter. The fear of lying under that bed waiting to see what would happen next stayed with me. It was a frightening time. This made me anxious about being at home alone at night for quite a while. It didn't help that Dad told me if you're home alone you should keep the lights off so people can't see which room of the house you're in.

Not long after this event, my parents left me at home alone all day and into the evening. I was so afraid, I had all the lights off so no-one knew where I was in the house, and a knife over my shoulder for protection. Crying and fearing for my life, I took half a dozen of every tablet I could find in the house so I could make the fear stop. Later that night, after my parents finally came home, my face swelled up and I got very sick. I confided in Mum and she took me to the hospital where they put a tube into my stomach to induce vomiting. I honestly don't remember much of this evening, but I do remember Mum wanting me to talk to the pastor at the church she started going to because she thought I might be depressed. I wasn't depressed but I couldn't tell Mum why I'd taken the pills. It was impulsive, I just wanted the fear and pain to stop.

At the end of this extremely difficult year, we went on a family camping trip. Dad liked to make sure we were comfortable so we had a 12-volt fridge, 12-volt TV, and the best tents and mattresses money could buy. I went fishing with my parents in the tinny we had attached to the roof of the car. We caught 52 flathead and of course Mum's was the biggest! While we were fishing, Mum and Dad started talking about how generally things weren't great and perhaps it would be fun to buy a boat and sail off into the sunset. This sounded very attractive to both of them, and they talked about it a lot more throughout this trip. While Dad could be a very difficult man, at times he could also be very entertaining and charismatic as he was always so convinced of his superiority. This delusion of superiority occasionally came crashing down in comical ways! During this particular holiday, he brought some accelerant to help light the campfire. Dad always liked to do things bigger and better than everybody else so he couldn't just start the fire in a normal way and it couldn't be any normal fire. It had to be the best campfire around.

This night, Dad retrieved the small metal can of petrol that was stored in the back of the crew cab ute and walked it over to the fire pit. As he began to pour the petrol over the wood, Mum commented, "That might be a little bit too much just to start a fire."

Dad laughed off her comments, "Don't be so silly – leave the fire to me."

He walked the petrol can all the way over to the other side of the camp to make sure it was out of the way, replaced the lid and walked back to the fire pit. He stood in front of the fire pit opposite this fuel can, lit a match and threw it on the wood. With a whoosh, the flames flew up high enough to singe the hair on his eyebrows, a trail of flames began to track from the fire pit across the campsite all the way to the metal can, the flame hit the top of the metal can and it exploded into flames, flying up high into the air like a rocket, dropping down nearby. We were in uproarious laughter as Dad struggled to maintain his composure! Whenever I recount one of these stories, I giggle because I'm reminded of Tim "the Toolman" Taylor's famous line from the popular 90s comedy show *Home Improvement*: "More power!"

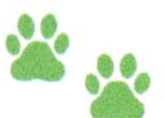

The school year started and the first term saw me failing Year 9 science and barely scraping through my other subjects. My parents were constantly being told school just wasn't for me. Truth be known, I was bored stiff and one of my teachers reminded me a lot of Dad. I understood the material but just couldn't be bothered learning it properly. I was constantly being bullied and couldn't see the point since I wasn't very bright anyway. Somewhere in the second term, we had a school ball, which I was miraculously allowed to attend despite my truancy and recurrent bad behaviour. I bought a beautiful pink dress and some white court shoes. I planned to meet up with my friends, ditch the ball, buy alcohol and get rotten drunk. Mum dropped me off at the ball, talking about how beautiful I looked and how much fun it would be, and I dutifully entered the hall as if I was going to stay until she picked me up later that night. I had other plans! My friends and I left as soon as we possibly could, got an older friend to buy alcohol for us, and sat in a nearby park drinking until it was time to go back to be picked up. I had been drinking and smoking, I was terrified Mum would be able to tell, but she didn't seem to notice and I went to bed thinking I got away with it.

The next day at school, my illusions would come crashing down. One of the teachers noticed we were gone and one of the other students had been caught, so we were now all in trouble. I would be one of the last students at this school to get the cuts. This was an old-fashioned form of corporal punishment, and it was brutal. A bamboo cane was slapped hard across your hands, both on the palms and then across the back of your hands over the knuckles. It definitely hurt, but by now physical punishment meant nothing to me. They called my parents in to have a meeting about the future of my schooling given that I was essentially failing, academically, socially and personally, to meet any of their expectations. After this meeting, it was agreed I would be pulled out of school to avoid expulsion. I was a couple of months shy of my 14th birthday and at the time you couldn't leave school until you turned 14. However, my parents were aware things weren't getting any better for me at school. My father firmly believed that I'd learn more from the "school of hard knocks" as he called it.

Two months before my 14th birthday, I stopped attending school and went to work in my mother's business full-time. When I turned 14, my parents applied for and received my formal exemption from school. I was so grateful for my Dad's attitude around school and for my ability to get out of this horrible cycle of bullying, academic failure and stress. I was working full-time, nine- or 10-hour days, bringing home $80 a week for myself. The rest was going to my parents for board and lodgings, but I didn't care. I was still better off.

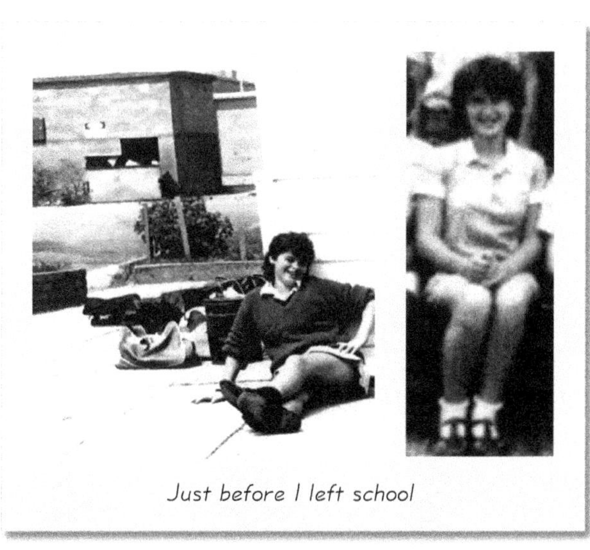

Just before I left school

My parents were still talking regularly about this pipe dream of buying a boat and sailing off into the sunset. Somewhere between my leaving school and the end of the year, they decided it was time to bite the bullet and sell up! Dad found his dream boat on someone's property somewhere in Victoria and convinced Mum it was a good idea to sell all our possessions, buy this boat, do it up and sail off into the sunset. They arranged to sell the house and then organised to have an auction of all our possessions. While I was excited at the prospect of this new adventure, I just couldn't be present when they auctioned off our private possessions. Absolutely nothing was sacred. Things were always disposable when it came to Dad so absolutely everything was up for sale in this auction. I spent the day shopping with a friend instead of attending the auction, returning only once it was over. Most of what we owned was gone, the house was bare and no longer our home. I was keen to go on the adventure. Once everything had been sold, and the business had been wound down, we were all packed, ready to leave for Victoria. We were off to live in a shell of a boat held up by wooden struts on someone's property in rural Victoria.

It was February 11, 1987, just as we were due to leave for our new adventure, when I received some devastating news that shook my little world. A good school friend, and my old boyfriend's best mate, had fallen off a cliff to his death at a youth camp. This was my first experience with death. It was confronting, particularly at such a young age. I attended the funeral and it was beautiful. He was so loved. I can still see the packed church with so many people they were standing in the back. I recall the tears on everyone's cheeks, a coffin taking centre stage. There were flowers running down the edge of the aisles and atop the coffin that I could smell even from the back of the church. I felt a deep sadness for my old boyfriend and his mate's family. The funeral gave me the chance to mourn with my peers and to say goodbye to them before we headed off. After my friend's death, I spent time writing poetry as a kind of therapy for my loss and grief. This was the first time

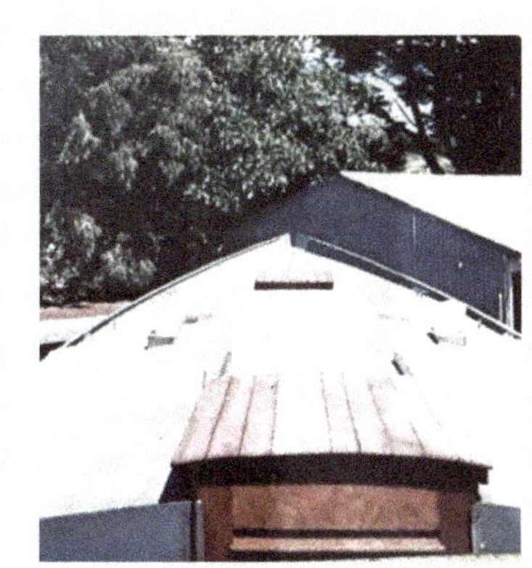

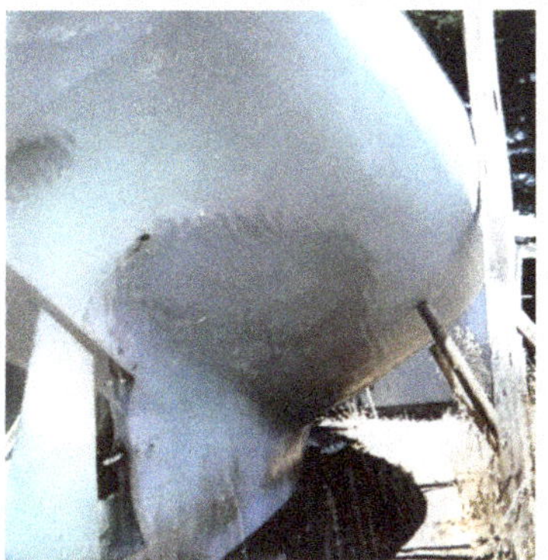

The boat in the paddock held up by wooden struts

I had put pen to paper as a coping strategy. Of course, I didn't realise at the time that's what it was, but I still use this strategy to this day.

We left on the boat from Devonport, arriving in Melbourne, picking up building materials that filled the ute to the brim. We drove for hours, with the gear stick bruising my right thigh each time Dad hit second gear, finally arriving at the shell of a boat in someone's back paddock in a tiny rural town of Northeast Victoria. As the sun set, we settled into our new home sweet home!

SILENCE

Hold your tongue, bite your lip, never speak a word of this

Secrets stay veiled behind smiles

A lifetime passes yet words never escape lips

Trapped in a ceaseless void of silence

Try to speak your truth, beware your tongue

Time passes, it's locked in the vault

On a solitary island of secrets, I sit

Tears flow as the silence deafens

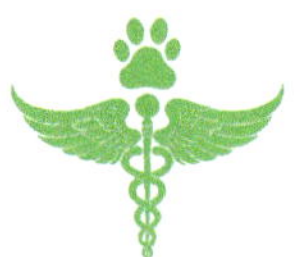

The following pages are intentionally blank. These pages are a tribute to anyone who has had to keep quiet or is unable to share their truth. Here I will sit with you in the silence, knowing the weight of this burden. You are no longer alone!

If reading this has caused you distress, please reach out to one of the following services in Australia. If you are outside of Australia, a simple Google search should help you find the support you need.

Key Mental Health Helplines in Australia at the time of printing:

- Lifeline (crisis support 24/7): call 13 11 14 or text 0477 13 11 14 for immediate support
- Beyond Blue (support for depression and anxiety): call 1300 22 4636 24/7 or chat online
- Suicide (prevention) 24/7 call back service: call 1300 659 467
- MensLine Australia (24/7 support): call 1300 78 99 78
- MindSpot (free online support for anxiety/depression/stress): call 1800 614 434
- FriendLine (for people feeling lonely): call 1800 424 287
- 1800RESPECT (24/7 support for people at risk of or experiencing family and domestic violence or sexual assault): call 1800 737 732
- 13YARN (a first nations crisis support line): call 13 92 76

These helplines are confidential and provide support for various mental health concerns. If you or someone you know is in crisis, please reach out to one of these services for help.

Remember, you are not alone, and support is available.

WHITE ANGEL

A rustling meow from deep in the bushes came
A helpless kitten emerging, as yet no name
Scooped up in caring arms, you're not alone
Could this be a happy ending, a loving home?
Looking deeply into your eyes, I promised you'd be just fine
However, decisions about your fate, sadly, would not be mine
I'm so sorry I couldn't keep you safe that day, my friend
This will be a failing I carry with me to the bitter end
Life snatched from your little paws without regard
Your short existence would be a lesson for me, so hard
No more would I trust, no more would I stay
Rest softly, white angel, I still remember you to this day

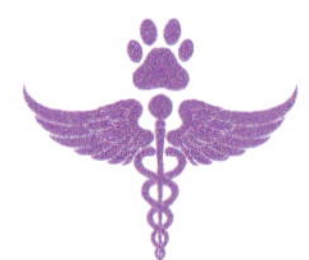

Victoria was a big change for us. We were now living in a tiny, rural town with rolling green hills and fresh air. With a population of around 2,500 people, a hotel and two local pubs were the highlights of the town. One of the advantages of moving around so much is you learn how to become very open; friendships are usually short and very intense. I made some great friends in Victoria. I was so relieved to not be at school, facing the relentless bullying and constant reminders of my intellectual inadequacies. It wasn't long before Dad reminded me I needed to contribute and, if I wasn't going back to school, I would have to go to work! I quickly reassured him I would rather work than go back to school any day, thank you very much. Within a week I had four part-time jobs, babysitting for two different families, cleaning and sweeping a garage. This was infinitely better than school. All my income went to support the family, aside from $10 per week. This was to be an ongoing allowance no matter how much money I earned and contributed to the family.

Most people would think this was unfair, but I finally felt useful as I was supporting my family. We had food every week as a direct result of the work I had been doing. However, it was all too much for my parents, having to ferry me around to four different jobs. It led to an ultimatum from Dad to get full-time work. I got an "almost" full-time job pumping petrol at the local service station and, as a compromise, also worked part-time at the local fish and chip shop. I felt great! I was enjoying the sense of stability and my personal contribution to the family made me feel valued.

Not long after I started working full-time, I met a kind young man and it wasn't long before I was smitten. Somehow, I got my parents to agree to let me go out on a date with him. It wasn't a real date, I don't feel like I ever really had one of those, but I was so excited to be doing something so "normal" and with my parents' consent, no less! Dad had relaxed his rules, reasoning if I was going to live in the adult world he would have to treat me like an adult. With my new relationship I started to feel like I was finally worth something to someone!

Dad always made it clear when others were around that I had little value. In fact, it always felt like Dad valued others over me in general. This kind of devaluation was a regular part of my relationship with him. I was still working almost full-time and working on the boat whenever I had time off. Both my parents had an excellent work ethic and expected nothing less when you helped them with any task. Not once did I consider doing anything other than manual labour in my life. This seemed to be the norm for my family; I wasn't smart enough to even consider other options. I was comfortable and happy with my work roles and didn't want for anything more.

Dad always had very high expectations regardless of the task at hand and held everyone to the same standard. There are a few distinct memories I have that involved some very manual tasks and Dad's unrelenting standards bordering on perfectionism. Dad was putting in the roof for the galley of the boat (that's what boaties call the kitchen) and needed to install insulation between the raw steel and the wooden panelling first. This was a task he delegated. I remember being in the enclosed space on a hot day, painting the glue on that steel hull, then on the back of the insulation bats and pressing them firmly into place. Very quickly I became dizzy and felt nauseated. I got the giggles and started to think I was getting high from the glue. Exiting the boat to get some ventilation, I stopped giggling and realised that this was serious! I could get quite sick from exposure to this glue. I spoke to Dad about how the glue was making me high, but his only concern was getting the job done! He told me to take frequent breaks and only bother him again when it was finished. There was a lot of giggling, lots of glue and not much work. I'm not sure how many brain cells were sacrificed for the task, but the job was done!

On another occasion, Dad asked me to put the thick protective coat on the bottom of the boat. Back in those days, people used an epoxy tar that was quite toxic both as an anticorrosive measure and a primer for the next coat called antifoul (a substance used to repel barnacles). I painted the entire undersurface of the boat, the part that would be under the water line, and then proudly showed him the finished product. He did his usual scrutinising and found multiple small holes where water could get in and cause electrolysis.

"That's not good enough. See these pock holes here?" he asked as he pointed at the tiniest of holes in the paintwork where you could *just* see the steel. "You need to fill these in. If a job's worth doing, it's worth doing properly!"

He handed me a tiny white spatula and a blue ice cream container filled with the thick, black tar that smelt just like the tar they used to fill potholes in the road.

"Come and get me when you're done."

I did this for a full day, trying to ensure I got every one of those stupid tiny holes because I knew he would inspect it closely. Apparently, I missed some and I was sent back to the drawing board with my blue ice cream container and spatula. This painful process went on for three full days.

He recurrently told me, "If a job's worth doing, it's worth doing properly, the first time!"

Those three days cemented in me a set of personal unrelenting and unrealistic standards that would cause me distress and anxiety for many years to come, with Dad's voice recurrently echoing in my head: *If a job's worth doing…*

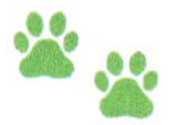

I was really enjoying my newfound freedom and foray into the adult world. I became sexually active fairly young in life. As always, Dad found out. He flew into a rage, as he had done so many times before, calling me all the disgusting names you can think of, lashing out and throwing things around. However, this time he did something different. He cried and then he threw me out. I was young, vulnerable, had no money and nowhere to go. I found somewhere to stay temporarily but I lived away from home for less than a month before the reality overwhelmed me. I begged my parents to let me move back home to the boat in the paddock, which of course Mum was keen for me to do. Dad agreed but with very strict conditions.

Essentially, I would do what I was told and it would not involve any boyfriends. I was initially compliant in the hope things would eventually settle down but I had no intention of staying compliant and I think Dad knew that. I thought I had satisfied his conditions, but Dad had other ideas. In his wisdom, he decided he needed to ship me off to learn some common sense. He would put me on a bus from Geelong to the Northern Territory to live with my maternal grandmother, the same woman my mother seemed to fear. What a great idea!

I was put on a three-day, three-night bus ride from hell with an eight-page letter from my mother, telling me she would come and get me as soon as she could. That letter was filled with all the reasons she loved me, all the good she saw in me and all the hope that things would be okay. She apologised for not being able to stop Dad from sending me away. I read it and cried until my eyes involuntarily closed, repeating this pattern each time I awoke. *Why can she never protect me from him?* I didn't understand the cycle of abuse at the time. I thought about what special torture living with Nana might bring. I don't think I slept properly for the entire trip. There was a lovely lady next to me on the bus who consoled me several times. On the last night I was restless and exhausted. I woke myself up, having accidentally rolled over and hit her in the face. I apologised profusely. I was barely sleeping, and the stress and fatigue were taking their toll.

Nana and Pop had long since divorced and Nana lived in a little unit on her own. To me, Nana was an old lady, set in her ways and of no interest to my teenage self. Mum and Dad never had a good story to tell about Nana, so I was scared. However, it wasn't at all what I expected. I spent three months living with her and it seemed I was now truly in the adult world, routinely attending over-30s clubs, dressing up, and free to drink and smoke. In my view, it felt like she paraded me around to everyone she knew as her "beautiful granddaughter". I felt like a piece of meat!

One night I found myself waiting for Nana on the edge of a dancefloor, dressed in an all-white, short, frilly, fancy dress she handmade for me, with white court shoes and lathered in makeup. I was sitting there waiting when this much older man sat down next to me. He whispered something in my ear. I couldn't hear him over the music. I thought he was telling me something about Nana, I leaned in closer so I could hear. Without notice, he put his tongue in my ear and I recoiled. I was disgusted and internally fearful of what would come next, but on the outside I giggled and smiled. I didn't know what else to do. He stayed in the seat next to me, with his arm around me, whispering in my ear and I was frozen! He asked me to go to some other club with him and I promptly said, "No, I'm waiting for my grandmother."

Nana finally came to the table, stating, "You've met my granddaughter then?" She obviously knew him and, while I'm not certain how he knew to talk to me, it felt very creepy. She chatted politely to this man for several more minutes as if she'd known him all her life. I quickly glugged down the last of my gin and tonic as I knew she was more likely to make me stay until my drink was finished. Yes, I was at an over-30s nightclub. Yes, I was 15 and yes, I had gin and tonic. I pretended to look unwell and asked to leave in the hope she would take me home. It was late and thankfully she agreed and we finally left. I had escaped this sleazy man who clearly knew who I was, which meant he had to have known I was much younger than him.

In my opinion, even though Nana never mistreated me, she certainly wasn't what I would consider a good influence on a teenage girl. I went drinking with friends frequently after this but never went back to the over-30s clubs. I don't think I ever felt like I could trust Nana to keep me safe again. I felt like she would throw me to the wolves if she had a chance of making herself look good. At the time, I didn't understand how risky this period of my life was. I was unsafe, underage and vulnerable. I count myself lucky that nothing untoward happened.

I got a full-time job in the jewellery department of a gift store and spent all of my income every week drinking and partying. Mum eventually caught a bus up to see me after three months to "save me" from living with Nana. I knew it had been risky but, when I look back now on that time, I realise it was the only real adolescence I ever had. I got to party, get drunk, wear whatever makeup and clothes I wanted, go out dancing all night, and spend all of my salary on alcohol without worrying for a second about the consequences. I hoped Mum meant it when she said she'd come back for me. I was so relieved to see her when she arrived one night that all I could do was cry and collapse into her arms. While I was in the Northern Territory, Dad launched the boat into the water, ready to put the rigging (the mast, etc.) on. I felt robbed of the opportunity to be present for the launch of the boat after spending nearly a year of my life supporting the family financially to achieve that very goal.

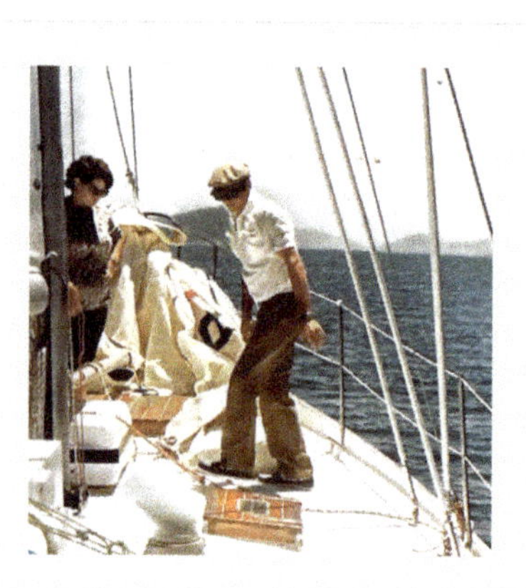
Living and sailing on the boat

Living with Nana had been a real education, but I was ready to move on.

Just before my 16th birthday, Mum and I left and headed back to the boat. I was back living with Mum and Dad on a boat, in the water, and somehow it seemed all was forgotten. While it seemed like everything was going well and I was finally starting to get along with Dad, it wouldn't be long before it all changed.

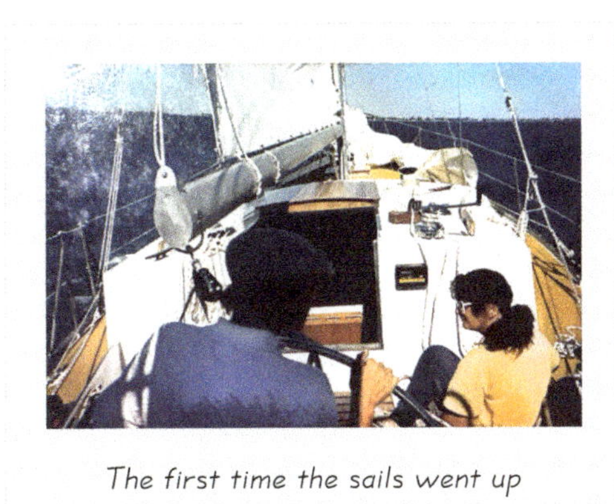

The first time the sails went up

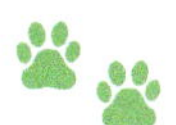

Sometime after we moved into the boat on the water, we went on a short trip away to look at a caravan park Mum and Dad were considering managing so that they could earn some extra money. I was now 16, still enjoying the adventure and in a relationship. While we were in this caravan park, I was out for a walk on my own when I heard meowing coming from the bushes. I pulled apart the foliage under the trees to see a single white fluffy kitten all by itself, crying for its mother. I looked everywhere but found no sign of a nest, other kittens or this kitten's mother. I couldn't leave it there to die, so I scooped the little kitten into my jumper, walked it back to the caravan we were staying in while tenderly reassuring it everything was going to be okay. My love for animals led me to volunteer at an animal shelter in Tasmania before I left school so I felt confident in my ability to take care of this kitten. It was pure white, tiny, helpless, and in need of compassion and support. When I got back to the caravan, only Dad was home, I showed him the beautiful little kitten I just found. He took it out of my hands and patted it, looking over its body from nose to tail, stroking it gently. It felt like I'd done the right thing and he would let me keep the kitten, if only long enough to take it to an animal shelter or find it a new home.

Out of nowhere, he suddenly said, "This thing is covered in lice."

His facial expression changed rapidly from tender and caring to angry and annoyed. I couldn't understand why he was angry, I knew we could just treat the kitten with a simple wash and remove the lice. Before I could even reason with him further, he looked me in the eye, coldly and angrily, and said to me, "This is all your fault," as he snapped this little kitten's neck right in front of me.

I was numb, frozen in place. I couldn't believe what had just happened but I knew from experience not to react.

It's hard to explain what it's like to see that absent look in a person's eyes while they end another living being's life in front of you. I don't think you can truly comprehend the instant sense of fear and threat you feel unless you have been faced with this degree of malice. I'd seen him do this to animals that he'd shot in the wild but not killed. In those instances, he killed them out of what I thought was compassion. This was different. He seemed to kill this kitten out of spite towards me. This was like being punched in the gut, or like he reached into my body, pulled out my heart and tore it into a million pieces. I couldn't react. I couldn't show weakness for fear of becoming the direct target of his anger. He proceeded to explain to me, "You should never have brought the damn thing home. I did it a favour. It was going to die anyway."

A part of me wondered if I could suffer the same fate if I upset him enough. Somewhere deep inside, my instincts told me how frightening this was and that I was no longer safe around this person, but I also felt so responsible. *This beautiful kitten would've been better off if it never met me. He is right. How stupid of me to bring this little kitten home. It's my fault it died!*

This was the first time I fully understood that Dad didn't have the capacity to empathise with another living creature. I started to shift my thinking a little, with the understanding there was something not quite right about this kind of behaviour. It was he who I now believed was abnormal. I still felt stupid and inadequate, but I also knew something about his behaviour was unhealthy and certainly risky for me to be around. Later that night, I sobbed quietly into my pillow for that beautiful little kitten and vowed never to bring another stray animal home again. We went back to the boat like nothing ever happened, but for me everything had changed.

I needed to get out, I needed to understand, I needed to know why he was like this. *Why does he hate me so much?* Within a few days of coming home from the trip to the caravan park, I would have an opportunity to ask him this very question. We were coming to blows constantly. In one of these frivolous arguments, I looked him straight in the eye and asked him, "Why do you hate me so much?"

"I don't know. I just do!"

Instead of scooping me up, reassuring me he didn't hate me, telling me how much he loved me, that was his response. This confirmed what I had known to be true my whole life: *My father hates me*. Sobbing, I quickly packed a bag and was stepping off the boat when Mum poked her head out of the hatch and said, "If you leave, I'm going with you!"

I didn't want to be responsible for an argument that may become physical or for Mum and Dad splitting up. Nothing more needed to be said. I gingerly turned around, stepped back on board the boat and started to plan another way to exit.

I would need to do it in a way that meant Mum wouldn't follow. The priority now was to get out and try to make a life for myself as far from Dad and his behaviour as I could get. I moved into a nearby caravan park with James, my new boyfriend at the time, soon after. I didn't have any significant possessions and my income was limited. The best I could do for the time being was to buy a three-man tent, an inflatable mattress, an Esky and a two-burner gas stove top. This was a new, humble little home and now I would live in a tent for three months until I could find work. It was a bitterly cold, extremely uncomfortable and meagre existence, but it was ours! Eventually we heard there was work grape picking in Mildura. We set off on this new little adventure, far away from Dad and all that he represented.

I was so excited to leave it didn't even occur to me how hard it might be to pick grapes in the searing heat. However, I certainly wasn't afraid of a little bit of hard work. This was going to be a new chapter in my life, one where I finally had some control. Picking grapes was hard, hot, sweaty work but I found ways to enjoy the days. The accommodation was dirty, dark, hot, and filled with pests and rat droppings, but it was infinitely better than a three-man tent. There was a bush toilet consisting of a bucket dug into a hole in the ground with a wooden square and a makeshift toilet seat over the top. We had to take it in turns emptying the toilet. When my turn came, I had several offers from the other workers to do it for me but this task didn't bother me at all. It was just a little bit of smelly, hard work. I was surrounded by fun-loving, interesting people and I was free to do what I wanted, within reason, all day. I had a deep sense of freedom and the constrained, harsh, strict environment of my home felt like a distant memory. Unfortunately, it was only a few months before it became clear to me the income wasn't enough to survive off, so I headed back to what was familiar, back to Mum and Dad. *What was I thinking? I can't survive on my own!*

I didn't recognise nor understand my father's narcissistic behaviours and the hold they had over me in terms of decision making and independence. Despite feeling liberated from the tight sense of control he always had over me and his volatility, I still returned repeatedly.

This just demonstrates the psychological pull of a controlling, abusive person in these kinds of relationships. The true strength of someone like my father lies in their uncanny ability to make everyone around them believe their narrative. He was so certain in his conviction that I would never make anything of myself that I, and many people around me, believed it.

BUB

So excited you're finally coming, this wasn't the first try
I just can't wait to meet you, to hear your first cry
I can feel you growing stronger and bigger each day
While I rub my belly, contemplating the first word you'll say
I already feel like I know you, your personality so free
Wondering what your future will be like, what you'll want to be
In anticipation, the first of many contractions begins
As I giggle on the laughing gas the midwife grins
Gran waits patiently, looking a bit weathered and worn
Then the time finally comes for you to be born
You entered this world in your own time, no hurry to come
That was fine by me, I was just so proud to be your mum
I'm so pleased to have you in my life, my beautiful baby boy
Waking up to your little face each day is my greatest joy
From now on you would be my priority number one
My heart full, you brought so much love and fun

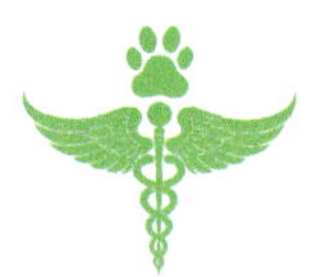

Going back, things weren't much better with Dad. I secured a job as a breakfast cook at a local motel, and I helped as Mum and Dad got the boat ready to "sail off into the sunset" as they dreamed. Not long after returning, James and I bought a caravan and, with Dad's help, a car to tow it. We took off up the east coast of Australia, travelling as far as Rockhampton. It was here where I first started to consider training in some kind of trade so I could earn a regular income. I applied for a chef's apprenticeship at a restaurant in Rockhampton, but my application was unsuccessful. I don't think I expected anything less. My father always told me how stupid I was and this was just confirmation.

The combination of my fear of failure and completely unrealistic standards for success prevented me from trying anything else for a long time to come. My parents sailed up the coast, arriving in a little place in Sydney affectionately known as The Puddle to the Pittwater locals. They proposed I come and join them, save up together and go sailing with them. This adventure sounded too good to be true. We sold the caravan and, with all we owned now in the car, arrived in Pittwater to join them. Some would say it was an omen that only two days into my time there the rusty old V8, with its broken exhaust, parked between two Mercedes sedans, was stolen with all my belongings in it, including CVs, written references, clothes, shoes, right down to toiletries. This would be a fresh start all right!

Almost a year of living, working and saving in Pittwater was indeed a great adventure! We met lots of new, exotic people from different parts of the world and partied with most of them. We had what we called progressive dinners where you would go from one boat to the next, having a different course each time, finishing off with cocktails on the final boat. Mum and I got work in a local fruit shop, getting paid well and working long hours to save for this elusive sailing trip. We were working hard and all my earnings were being put into the "kitty", as Dad called it, for our future adventures together. At one of these rather outrageous beach parties, one of the foreign nationals from New Zealand treated us to a traditional hāngī. He enlisted us all to help dig the large hole in the sand, place the hot coals in there and wrap the meat in foil, covering it all back up with sand. You could smell the meat cooking while we all sat around, shared stories, laughed and drank.

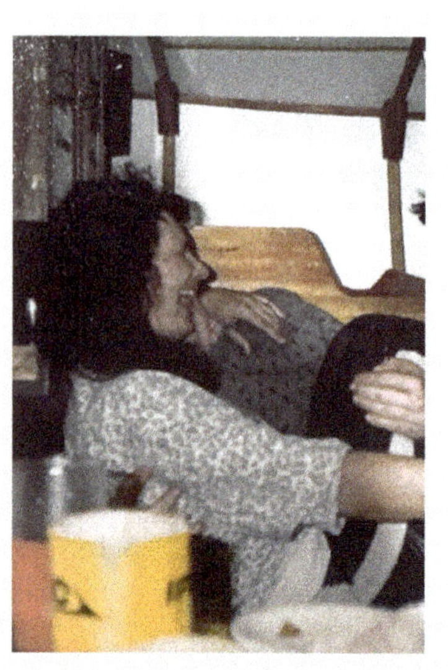
Mum partying on the boat

As we were leaving this party, Mum and I noticed a gentleman who'd left much earlier was sitting in his dinghy, rowing frantically on the sand, trying desperately to get to his boat. He looked puzzled when we pointed out to him he wasn't even in the water! We were almost wetting ourselves with laughter trying to explain what was going on to this drunk gentleman who barely spoke a word of English. We gave him a lift back to his boat, ensuring he got below deck safely before we left. At one of these parties, at the age of 17, I was offered cocaine by a reveller. I declined, with Dad's voice once again echoing in my head: *You don't have to pour battery acid on yourself to know it's going to burn.*

At some point it became clear it was unlikely anyone would end up going on this round-the-world, dream sailing trip Dad kept talking about. All my income had gone to the kitty while I was there. I began to want something different. I remembered what life was like when I was grape picking, how free I felt and how exciting that was to me. I wanted more. It was around this time, at 17 years of age, I got engaged. I chose my engagement ring and we had a little celebration at a local Chinese restaurant where Dad expressed how happy he was that I'd found such a good man in James.

One day, Dad and a few other people were sitting in the cockpit (the little enclosed pit at the back of the boat where the captain steers from) when Dad and I somehow ended up in a minor argument about something trivial, as we so often did.

Dad was angry and blurted out, "I don't know how you put up with this bitch."

In front of everyone. I was quite surprised he said that out loud, in front of other people. I waited for someone to speak up and defend me, but it didn't happen. It was just laughed off and the conversation switched to something completely unrelated. I now believe when this happens normal people are affronted, but they don't know what to say and the default is to try to keep the peace. But I wanted someone to stand up for me.

Stunned at Dad's disrespect, I went inside the boat and immediately started to pack. I was livid! Mum was trying to calm me down and convince me to stay but I knew I had to leave. While packing, all I could think was: *How dare he? How rude and in front of others.* I was humiliated. Again, it felt like no-one stood up for me. Again, it felt as though Dad's behaviour went unchallenged. I just couldn't keep doing this to myself! I was learning this was a pattern that came from the cycle of abuse experienced in my childhood, and I needed to stop exposing myself to this pattern. I was also learning I was often the one who stood up to him and the constant fighting was tiring. I left the boat the next morning and moved to Geelong to live with my now fiancé, James. I demanded my parents send me back the money I contributed to the kitty and they did end up sending me enough to make a fresh start.

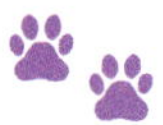

Geelong was a great change for me. I worked at a local bakery and despite the early hours I loved it! We found a cute little unit that technically didn't permit pets but I wanted a little Chihuahua, so I got Wingnut, and I bought a horse that was agisted at the previous owner's property. I loved animals and just wanted to be surrounded by them whenever I could. I was making friends and quickly settled into this newfound domestic bliss.

However, as a result of my unhealed trauma I was insecure and my mind always took me to: *I'm not good enough, I'm stupid, uneducated, no-one will ever really love me and if they do they will eventually leave me anyway!*

I would have been around 18 when I got the next "we need you to come and help" message from Mum and Dad. They had sailed the boat up the east coast of Australia all the way to the Gold Coast, then experienced some relationship difficulties. Mum told me she just returned from spending some time away and they were trying to reconcile. They decided to sell the boat and move back into a house on land. As part of the sale, they traded the boat for a house and some money, allowing them to buy a small business delivering bread to local stores. They resolved to stay together but would need to go on a trip away to reconnect. Mum asked me if I would manage their business for them while they attempted to salvage their marriage.

As I had always done, I dropped everything and went up to Queensland to help them. After spending a few weeks teaching me how to run their small business, they left on their trip away and, suddenly, I was there managing a small business at 18! I loved the management side of the business, including the accounts. My parents were supposed to be gone for a few weeks, but they were gone for months. I didn't mind. The business had good cash flow, so money wasn't an issue and I really enjoyed myself. Sadly, one day Dad contacted me to tell me he wanted to sell this little business. I was upset and a bit disappointed, having uprooted my entire life to be here, but had loved every minute of the adventure. Being involved in my parents' lives was never boring, that's for sure! I put together a contract of sale, advertised and sold the business for them. I felt so capable running this little business and thought *perhaps I found something I might be good at in future*?

With the business sold and my parents on their way back, this meant I would be living with them again. I reasoned: *I'm older now, this time will be different*. Dad was always on the lookout for the next big deal so we didn't stay put for long. He sold the house and bought a rundown business in Far North Queensland. There was a promise of work in this business and the new dream started to become a reality. Once again, I uprooted and followed my parents' dreams, setting up home with James in a caravan park. It was small but cosy and it was home. I always wanted to be a young mum so I could relate to my children better than my parents related to me, something James and I seemed to agree on, so this would be the next focus in life.

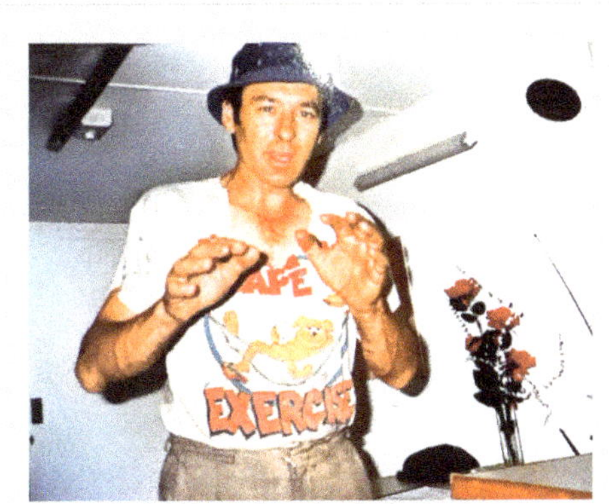

Dad's classic "look out" stance while handing over the business

I started trying to fall pregnant and at age 18 I was expecting my first child. I was so excited! This child was planned, would be so loved and wanted. I had a whole future mapped out for my little family. At eleven weeks I started to get some bleeding, which I read could be normal so I wasn't particularly worried. I went to the doctor and she booked me for a scan. My little baby was visible on the screen. I could see the little outline of a tiny human. For a moment I was excited until the sonographer interjected coldly, and I will always remember her words, "I'm sorry but there's no heartbeat. Your baby is dead."

I don't think I even knew what a miscarriage was or considered that this could happen to me. My young mind couldn't process what was happening.

The doctor allowed me to go home and wait to see what happened. As the days drew on, I started to bleed very heavily and had to go to the hospital. I was passing large, tennis ball sized clots, having to have them removed with a speculum (a large, beak-shaped instrument they insert into the vagina) and all the humiliation that came with it. I had low blood pressure and they decided I needed to go to surgery to have a curette, a procedure I was told would remove the remains of my baby as they were making me bleed.

"My baby died," I sobbed as I relayed the situation to Mum, with Dad in the corner of the room. "I have to have surgery to remove what's left to stop the bleeding."

Mum was visibly worried reassuring me the best she could, "It'll be all right, Jo, they know what they're doing." One of the nurses came in to do their checklist before surgery and I could hear Mum and Dad talking in the background. Dad wasn't consoling Mum and all I heard him say was, "She's probably faking it anyway. She's always so emotional, overdramatising everything. I don't think there's anything wrong with her."

How could he be so insensitive? How could he not believe me when I'm being taken to theatre? This kind of minimisation was a constant feature of my relationship with Dad and it seemed no-one around him would ever call him out on this behaviour. This type of language – "she's being dramatic, she's so emotional" – still triggers me to this day.

I was *very* emotional and wanted to clean myself up. They let me have a shower but I had to have someone with me because I had low blood pressure. I was desperate to wash off the day and feel better. None of my family were there so a male nurse accompanied me into the shower.

I remember feeling exposed, violated and vulnerable, and breaking down in tears of trauma and embarrassment as I felt the warm blood drip down both my inner thighs and heard the *plop* of a large clot falling into the water in the shower well below me. That beautiful male nurse comforted me. He was so respectful, so empathetic and so human. I was incredibly lucky to have him caring for me and, as I left the hospital, I made sure he knew how much he'd helped me at an incredibly difficult and lonely time in my life. His compassion and care was inspiring, and it made me want to help others the way he had helped me.

I don't recall my family being there when I got back from theatre, but I was in a bit of a haze. When I was finally able to sit up, I was all alone. Recovering from the miscarriage felt very lonely. As is the case with any significant loss, I think even if others are present, if it's happening to you and your body it's something you experience alone. Nobody seemed to want to talk about it, so it was like it never happened. I think there's a lot of personal discomfort for people around pregnancy loss and they tend to avoid talking about traumatic events so they don't upset the person who experienced it. I'm not built that way! I needed to talk about it. So, I talked *at* the people around me, leant on Mum, cried and mourned until I felt like I could move forward.

I was still trying to fall pregnant. The doctor had advised that after a miscarriage can be the most fertile time and within three months I was pregnant again. I was excited and scared at the same time. I decided not to tell anyone about it after reading that miscarriage is most common in the first three months of pregnancy. Counting the days, and crossing my fingers it would all go well this time, I waited until I was three months pregnant then shouted to the world that I was having a baby! I was so excited at the thought of becoming a mother, of nurturing another little human being into adulthood. I had so much love to give and I started giving it while my baby was still in the womb. I would talk to the baby and affectionately named it Bub. I would sing to them, rub my belly and proudly announce to anyone who would listen my baby would be here soon. I couldn't wait to be a mum.

I had an uncomplicated pregnancy, going well over my due date, and moved into a little flat on the Sunshine Coast in preparation for the birth of this little baby. I started labouring 72 hours before my son, Eliot (Eli for short), was born. I went to the hospital but they kept sending me home, saying it was too early. Eventually I was admitted as I needed to have an epidural for the pain. It didn't matter what I had to do. Somehow, I knew I could get through it. I would do anything for this child!

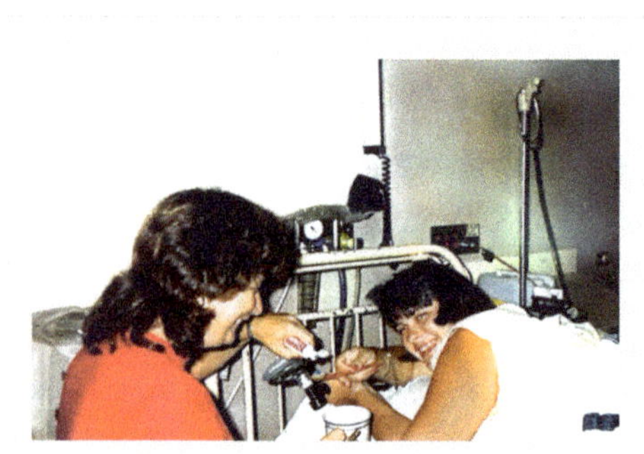

On laughing gas in labour

Eliot was born at 4.15pm on August 15, 1991. While they spent an hour or so stitching me up, I stared lovingly into this little perfect creature's eyes! I looked at his skinny little legs, and his tiny fingers and toes. I was smitten! I just knew this was what I was put on this Earth for! Everyone was equally enamoured with our new little man except for Dad. Mum forced Dad to come and meet Eliot and he initially refused to hold him, stating he was too fragile. Mum insisted he hold him and we got a picture of Dad holding his first grandchild. After a few hours they took him to the special care nursery because he was having a little bit of trouble with his breathing. It had been a marathon few days. Exhausted, I fell asleep. When I woke up I realised it had been seven hours since he was born and I was alone. He wasn't with me. *Where's my baby? Is there something wrong with him?* Flustered, I demanded to see him and they brought him straight back to the ward, relieving a brief period of intense panic.

I was so grateful to finally have this baby in my arms, I couldn't lose him. A lovely midwife taught me how to breastfeed and gave me all sorts of troubleshooting tips. I wanted to go home straight away and insisted I would get more rest at home. They spoke to the doctor and arranged for me to go home on their newly developed early discharge plan. This would involve a midwife coming out to the home every day for a week to check on us and my wounds. This was a wonderful program and I was so happy to be going home with this beautiful baby! We were a family; I was so proud and I loved this baby so much.

I was absolutely thriving as a 19 years young, first-time mum. I loved every minute of taking care of this fragile, dependent, beautiful child. My heart was absolutely bursting with love and affection! I started to realise this was the first time in my entire life I felt competent at something. I just knew I was going to be a good mum and that I could take care of this child no matter what happened. However, the more I thought about his future, the more I considered as he got older my lack of formal education may impact on my ability to help him with his schoolwork. *If he has an uneducated, unintelligent mum, will that impact on his education?* I started to think about what this might mean and if I was going to be serious about being a good mum, I might need to get an education myself. I didn't even have a Year 9 education!

I couldn't see how to achieve this but I started to consider it would be necessary at some point to improve my own education, to become a better mum and provide better opportunities for my children. I worried about this a lot and at times it even kept me up at night. I didn't even have a driver's licence as my father's words were always playing on a loop in my head: *You're too stupid! Don't be so silly! You'll never amount to anything anyway. You're stupid, subordinate, a waster* (meaning a waste of time), *useless.*

I didn't even try most new things for fear of failing at something. However, being a mum gave me a newfound courage to challenge this. The determination and unrelenting standards handed down from Dad were somehow in conflict with these beliefs of inadequacy. It was a constant, exhausting internal battle from the moment my son

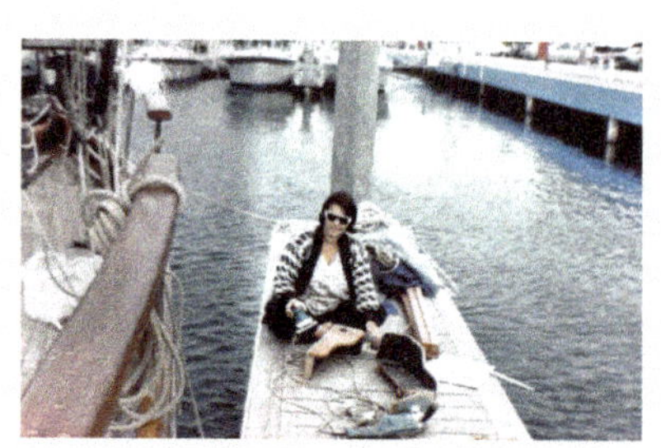

Sanding the light runner, six months pregnant

was born. Even if I was stupid, I would just have to work harder to overcome this to help my kids and create the life they deserved! I knew I could work hard – that was never a problem. *Perhaps you can overcome stupid with hard work.* I was too scared at this point to do anything about it but it sat, marinating, in my brain.

I tried several times to get my learner's licence while in this little flat, failing the test not once, not twice but seven times! So afraid of failure, so nervous I would shake and get uncontrollable diarrhoea before each attempt. I finally gave up on the notion of passing this test and conceded that I was in fact stupid, like Dad had always told me! *Who fails their driving test seven times?* I was 21 years old before I attempted the driving test again, this time at the insistence of my beautiful mum who reminded me if anything happened to Eliot, I needed to be able to drive him to get help. I could drive and I had raced go-karts so I was a capable driver. I had just been so nervous about failing the test that I failed every time. This time was different; I was doing this for my child, not for me! Miraculously I passed the learner's test and then the formal driving test (in a manual car, no less) and was finally licensed to drive!

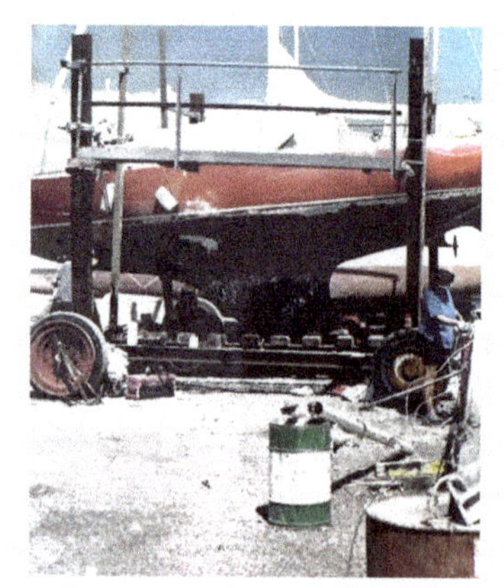

Sanding the mast of one of my own boats, just before I was admitted for anaphylaxis

The little voice in my head that told me how useless and stupid I was reared its ugly head every time I took the wheel, so I deferred to others whenever I could to keep Eliot safe from my incompetence! Mum had also brought to my attention that I seemed to apologise all the time, even when I wasn't responsible for something. If someone else ran into me or hurt me, I would lower my head and say, "Sorry."

This was the result of that internal negative dialogue. I felt in the way no matter where I was or what I was doing. I always felt like the scapegoat for Dad and I had learnt to shrink away and make myself invisible to stay safe, and avoid being kicked in the backside or slapped over the back of the head!

We spent a lot of time around my parents throughout Eliot's young life and my Mum was very close to him. Dad was very distant and treated him the way he treated me when I was young, like he was in the way. I was conscious of limiting his exposure to my dad. James and I bought a boat and were living on this in the hope it could be renovated and sold for a profit. This was a desperate attempt to get ahead using the only skills I knew. We bought a few boats, renovating them and selling them. Dad became quite unwell while Eliot was a baby, requiring a triple bypass operation, which changed my parents' plans a little. It also changed my perspective. I wanted to spend time with my dad and get to know him while I could. I wanted to enjoy things while I still had them. I was in North Queensland with a boat in a boatyard, trying to

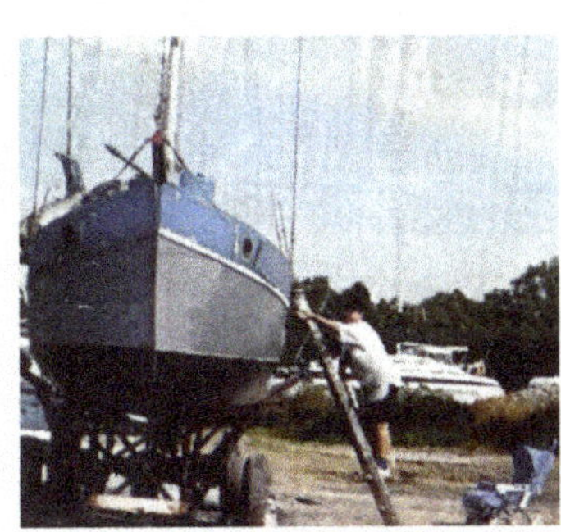

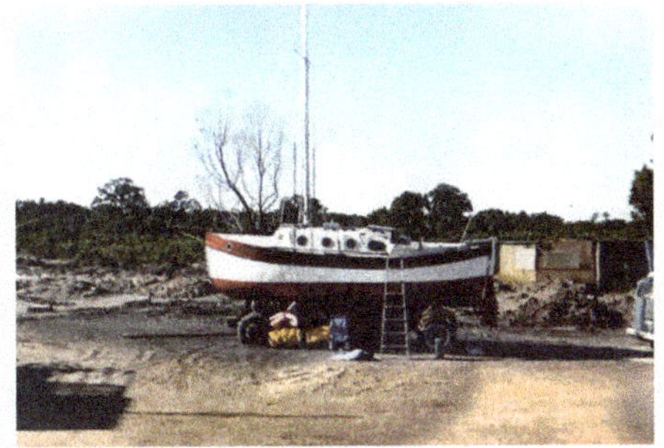

Working on the first boat I ever bought and renovated

figure out next steps, while providing support to Mum and Dad while Dad recovered from his operation.

When Eliot was 18 months old, James and I got married and Eliot was the ring bearer. I was delighted that he might have memories of this day, like I did with my parents' wedding. I tried to have some time away but, after only three days, I missed Eliot so much it was hard to relax. This was the longest I had ever left him with family, and I felt the urge to get back to him. Throughout my children's young lives, I had extreme anxiety around leaving them with others; I always worried that what happened to me as a child may happen to them.

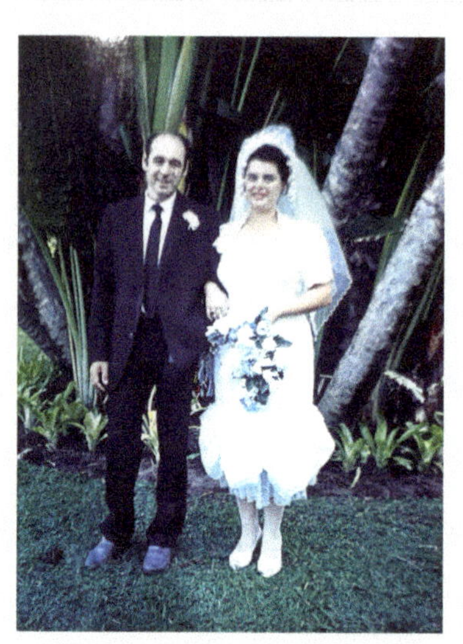

Dad walking me down the aisle

While living in the boatyard, I met a couple, Bill and Nang. They owned the boat across from us and Eliot would smile and say hello to Nang every time she went past, befriending her from the cockpit. Nang was from Malaysia. She was gregarious, generous and fun-loving. I struck up an immediate friendship with Nang and we did all sorts of fun things together. She was the first female adult friend I ever really had, and I loved her company. She absolutely adored children, loved to cook for people and we got along very well.

Mum and Dad took off on their new adventure to New Zealand. We were on our own little adventure in the boatyard with my newfound friends! I partied long into the evenings with Nang and she shared wild stories from her homeland and sailing adventures. I also shared many of my traumatic childhood stories and the difficulties with my dad with my new best friend. It was a lovely time and Nang and I became very close.

That was, until I got the all-too-familiar call: "We need you to come to New Zealand to help us get the boat ready to sail. We can't do it without you."

Once again, I uprooted our lives, leaving behind the lovely little boat and new friends, to go on my parents' next adventure. This time, it would be much more than I bargained for!

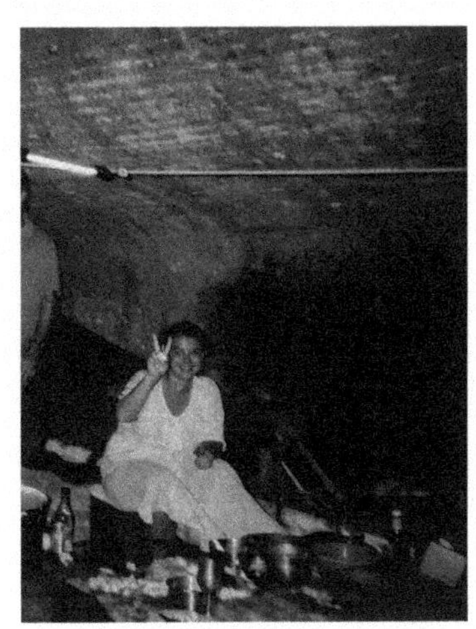

Barbecue with Nang under a boat in the boatyard

When we arrived in New Zealand, I was still breastfeeding Eliot and I was violently ill with some form of gastroenteritis. Mum and Dad were working at Whangarei while I stayed on the boat tied up to the pylons in Auckland. So much for helping them – I was of absolutely no use. I was so sick with nausea, diarrhoea and vomiting. I had to row over to the shore to go to the toilet, with Eliot in a special backpack, and ended up just staying onshore for hours at a time because I needed to use the toilet up to 17 times a day. I was unwell like this for a week. I didn't go to a doctor. And every day, they got up, went to work and left me there. Thank goodness I was young, fit and healthy before that struck. By the time I could eat properly and felt a bit better, it was clear to me that Mum and Dad were having relationship issues again.

Mum wanted to go home to Australia. She said Dad wouldn't give her the airfare and that's one of the reasons she asked me to come. Mum had decided to leave Dad – he knew it, and he was using financial control to stop her from leaving. This was no surprise to me. This had happened many times before, with Dad having absolute financial control in the relationship. I had a long conversation with Mum and she decided to leave him and come back on the plane with me. I also wanted to go home as it had been an awful time for me. After three months she had what she needed and we boarded a plane using some money Dad had asked Mum to pay a bill with. She left a note for him to read when he got home.

Mum was so relieved to be able to leave, having said she was frightened of how it would have ended if I hadn't been able to help. Dad could be a scary man, she had been physically threatened and even harmed by him many times before, so I didn't doubt this could have ended badly for her. I did, however, feel dreadful about how we left and Dad took it very badly. He was angry but mostly with me for helping Mum, and with Mum for leaving him with a bill to pay, which I didn't realise had something to do with the boat. Once the bill related to the boat was paid off and the boat was seaworthy, Dad set sail for Australia.

The boat finally arrived in the harbour close to the boatyard where we were living at the time. Mum and I watched as it motored in and anchored, and then she left. Dad stayed on my boat in the boatyard for a couple of nights. There were times when he was out of radio contact so we were all grateful when he made it safely back to Australia with the boat intact. It had been a stressful time. I breathed a sigh of relief. We were all now back on Australian soil, safe and sound. At 2am on the second night after he returned, we were awoken by a knock on the hull of our boat. I went out to see two policemen asking after Dad. He was taken to the station as he'd brought the boat into the country without paying import duty. We spent hours at the police station and Dad was fuming the entire time. They threatened to impound the boat, but he managed to arrange a grace period to get the money together.

The boat was taken out of the water and put in the same boatyard where we lived. Mum and Dad were attempting to reconcile, and it seemed like they would be getting back together. As she owned half the boat, they had to resolve this import duty problem together. But the drama around the boat was probably the nail in the coffin for the relationship. While all this was happening Mum and Dad's relationship again became strained. It was around this time that I introduced Dad to my good friend, Nang. She mentioned how "sexy" he was and I told her to stop being so silly and that was gross. *He's my dad!*

Dad also mentioned that she was very attractive. I told Dad she was my best friend and absolutely off limits! But they began an affair that would end both their marriages, leaving me feeling sandwiched firmly in between. I didn't realise it at the time, but this had a lasting impact on friendships for me. I was much more guarded and avoided getting too close to people. I felt both of them had betrayed me. Much later in life, a former medical colleague once said to me, "I really wanted to be your friend, but you were so hard to reach."

I had learnt from experience that the harder you are to reach, the less likely you are to be hurt!

BABY GIRL

I knew I wanted you well before you came along
Now you're on your way, my heart is filled with song
A little girl, all that's needed to feel complete
My love for you grew with your every little heartbeat
You would enter the world in an environment of calm and peace
When you arrived the longing could finally cease
Your warm and loving eyes met my gaze
Your arrival filled lives and brightened days
"Beautiful baby girl, I vow to love you for all time"
I whisper quietly with your tiny little hand in mine
I wonder what adventures we'll have, what sort of life you'll plan
I promise to be there to protect and love you as best I can
As you gently rest in my arms and fall asleep
I'm reminded of all the promises I must keep
Your every breath now a source of joy so pure
I know you will always be loved, of that I am sure

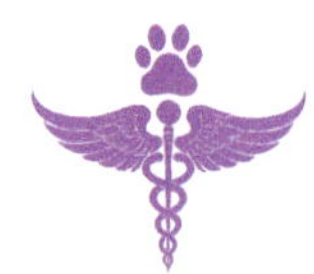

While Dad and Nang were starting their tryst, and with all the changes happening in both our lives, Mum and I decided we needed to do some personal development. We found a course called Positive Living at the local Technical and Further Education (TAFE) facility that didn't require any qualifications. We reasoned that we could use some positivity in our lives and, since neither of us was brave enough to do anything like this on our own, we decided to do this little six-week course together.

We were both very nervous as neither of us had so much as a high school education and TAFE was where smart people went to learn. We expressed our concerns to Mindy (the lovely lady who facilitated this course) and she reassured us anyone could do it, regardless of background. Mum left school when she was 15 due to ongoing illness, so this was as new to her as it was to me. The course was held in the evenings and as we arrived at our very first session there was an excitement neither of us had felt before, a sensation that this could be life-changing!

Mindy taught us all about our nervous systems and negative inner critics. She challenged us to eliminate negative self-talk, talk more positively about others and listen rather than overthink. She taught us about meditation and the power of positive thinking. She wasn't over the top or eccentric. She was well educated, and what she said and asked us to do had great power. Mum and I started to call each other out on negative dialogue and encourage each other to be better versions of ourselves. We started to believe we could do more, *be* more.

We also started to explore spirituality. We weren't religious and neither of us wanted to go to a traditional church, but we both wanted more of this 'positive living'. We felt better about ourselves and for the first time in my life I thought: *What if I could become something more than Dad told me I could be, more than even I expected?* We stumbled across a local spiritual church that espoused the same kind of acceptance, positive outlook and meditative practices as Mindy, and set about attending. We arrived for our first ever meeting at Eagle Lodge Spiritual Centre, run by a beautiful human named Ann Williams-Fitzgerald. In the carpark we watched as several relaxed, lovely people entered the facility and were hugged, one after the other, as they proceeded through the door. We both looked at each other and agreed that if they hugged us, we would leave and never come back! I'm quite sure we exuded the 'don't hug me' energy as not one soul tried to hug either of us.

They started the evening with a Native American tradition called the talking stick. Whoever had the stick had the floor and no-one could interrupt them as they spoke. It was so foreign to us to have to speak in front of others, let alone about ourselves. When that stick came to me, my stomach was churning like a raging sea. All the saliva in my mouth dried up and a lump bigger than Mount Everest developed in my throat. Holding my sweaty palms tightly around this 'talking stick', I swallowed that giant lump and introduced myself, stating, "My name's Jodi and I'm from here."

My voice was so quiet that someone asked me to repeat my name. "Sorry, it's Jodi," and then I quickly offloaded this stick to the next person.

It wasn't unusual for me to be so nervous. I had so little self-esteem that I regularly apologised for my very existence. The final part of the meeting was a meditation and we both found this really relaxing and positive. We stayed for a quick cup of tea and spent the whole drive back to the boatyard laughing about how we would never have come back if they hugged us, how scary that stick was, and sharing how much we enjoyed the experience. We continued to attend this spiritual church for around 18 months and developed some deep, meaningful relationships with some very positive people. This showed me another side of life. I started to gain confidence with the talking stick, started to feel more accepted by those around me and really bonded with Mum on a whole other level. I wrote and recited poetry, honed my meditation skills and developed an interest in any form of self-improvement that was presented. I had believed for so long that I was so defective that surely any self-improvement would be good. I was a sponge, soaking up this positive energy and the confidence that came with interacting with self-assured people.

Our time at Eagle Lodge will always hold special memories for me, both for the healing it gave me personally and for the special time I got to spend with my mother. However, this time was also special for another reason. I had been diagnosed with endometriosis and, after a laparoscopy to investigate what I called "my monthly massacre", I was told my fertility may be compromised. This led to the decision to try for a second child while I still could. Having two children was always the plan for our little family and it wasn't long before I was pregnant again. I was so happy to be pregnant and so excited to be bringing this little life into the world. I was also pleased this child would be born at a time when I had a more positive outlook.

However, it once again raised the concern in me that I wouldn't be able to help my children with their homework. I also broke my toe in the boat, which forced the realisation that living on a boat with two children, particularly when one is a newborn, was unlikely to very comfortable. We moved into a little house that was so rundown they scheduled it for demolition after we moved out. However, this was a temporary solution.

Computers were also starting to become mainstream around that time and I figured if I was ever going to get a "real" job, I would need to know how to use one.

At the age of 24, heavily pregnant, I took an introduction to computing class at the local TAFE. I had completed a TAFE course before and this one also had no entry requirements, so I reasoned I should be able to do it. I learnt how to turn on the computer, how to perform basic Excel functions and word processing. This course was extremely difficult and I felt very unintelligent and inadequate throughout, but still managed to pass it so it came with some sense of achievement.

Buoyed by this newfound sense of competency, I applied for an early childhood education certificate at TAFE, but my entry was declined. When speaking to them, they said that a Year 10 school leavers certificate was an essential entry requirement. I asked to see the course coordinator and, still heavily pregnant, pleaded with her, stating that even though I didn't have a school leavers certificate, I would try harder than anyone else and would be the "best student they ever had". All to no avail. They couldn't help me because I simply didn't meet the entry requirements and I left bitterly disappointed.

We moved into a lovely little three-bedroom house in the suburbs in preparation for the baby's arrival. I started to explore returning to high school to complete Years 11 and 12, but they also required a Year 10 certificate. I was talking to the local Centrelink branch and looking into every avenue I could find at the time, but it all had to go on the back burner because I had a baby to deliver!

Angelina (affectionately nicknamed Angie) entered the world at 9am on February 5, 1996 at a midwife-only birthing centre. I tried to make her birth as relaxed and calm as possible, with a CD playing rainforest sounds, and essential oils and meditation my preferred methods of pain relief, supported by the occasional puff on nitrous oxide. Having said that, there were several additional people at her birth, including James, Eliot, my mum, Anne from Eagle Lodge and the midwife. At the last minute, my dad also asked to come in. He had never seen a birth so I agreed. As strange as that sounds, it felt natural at the time. In some odd way, Dad seemed to acknowledge how difficult the birthing process was and I think it was a profound experience for him as there were complications after her birth. Angelina needed immediate support from the midwife before she could breathe on her own. I had no idea any of that was happening, I was blissfully unaware of the chaos.

Mum told me later that the room was silent as the midwife worked with Angelina, and the onlookers were afraid she wouldn't make it. Angelina had other ideas and, just as I turned around, she was pinking up and crying. I was just as in love with this beautiful girl as I had been when Eliot was born. I didn't think it was possible to have my heart swell with so much love a second time. Eliot had been amazing throughout Angelina's birth and continued to absolutely adore her. He helped me with her first bath and nappy change. It seemed that in his eyes, his little sister was just perfect. I had a complete family and it felt so good and so right!

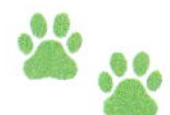

It was time to sell the little boat and permanently move onto land. Angelina was still a baby when we moved into a more comfortable house on a hill. When we went to look at this house, Eliot decided it was "magic" with its beautiful garden and special little rooms. This started a tradition of naming the houses we lived in. Eliot named this house "the magic house" and the kids thrived here, with the space, the garden and the special secret room Eliot found, which was really a formal dining room we never used.

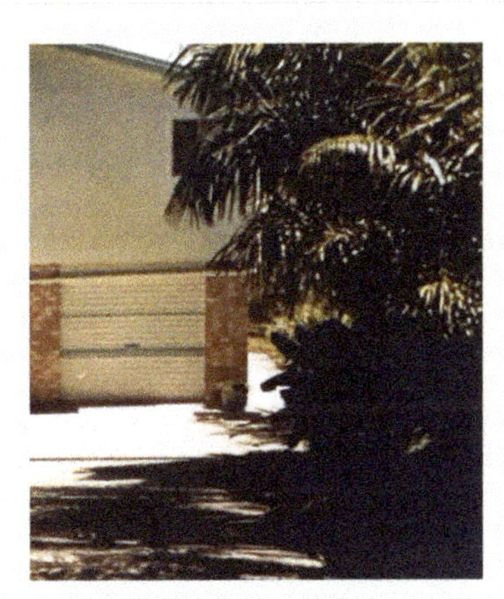

"The magic house"

Dad was determined to buy the boat from us but didn't have all the cash so he came up with one of his special deals. He was offering to trade the boat for what money he had and all his tools, which had significant resale value. I was happy to agree as the family was quite settled in "the magic house". The day came for the handover of all the money and tools. I was at Dad's house collecting things when Angie needed a feed. I was still breastfeeding at the time, so I got her out of the car seat capsule and fed her at his dining table. While I was feeding Angelina, Dad became very agitated and asked me when I would be signing the lease. I was confused as there was no lease associated with this deal. He explained that he wanted me to take over the lease on the house he was renting, with rent of $650 a week. I told him I would never have agreed to this, there was no way I could afford it with two children. He was adamant we would have to take over this house lease and started to escalate. The anger and the look in his eyes were very familiar to me. *I need to get out of here, now!* I started to get Angelina ready to go because I knew what came next. As I stood up to put her in the car seat capsule, Dad lunged forward with his fist flying towards me. Thankfully, he didn't make contact but it was clear that he was angry and I felt very threatened.

I bundled Angelina up and quickly headed to the car. Pulling out of the driveway I heard him yell threateningly at me, "I have friends in low places, you know. You never know when they might come around in the middle of the night. You never know when they might come for you!"

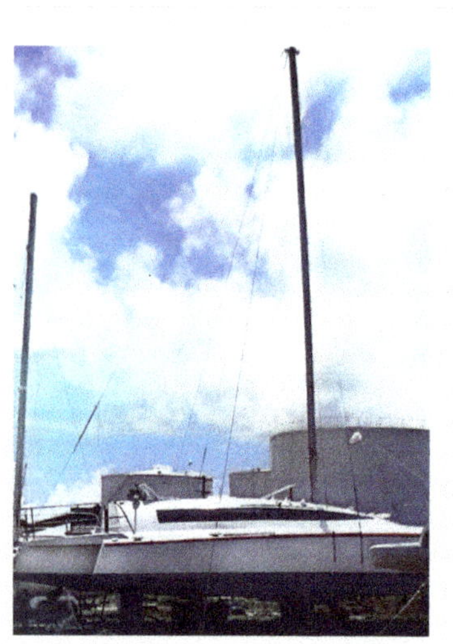

The boat Dad bought

I was genuinely afraid for a week or so. I knew Dad was capable of violence and was pretty sure he had some fairly sketchy friends in the past. I kept the doors locked in the house and became hypervigilant, checking the house for a couple of nights. When things had settled down, Dad finally paid the cash and realised he would have to see out the lease on his rental himself. It later became clear there were issues with the council. He was finding it hard to work on his cars there and that's why he wanted to get out of the lease, though he had never communicated that to me. This was a timely reminder of how volatile he could be and how important it was to minimise my children's exposure to him and his behaviour.

"The magic house" was just one of many houses we lived in, but it was here that the trajectory of our lives would change forever. One day I was at home with the kids when there was a letterbox drop with all the routine junk mail. Poking out the side of the pile, in between all the glossy shopping brochures, was a hand-folded black and white leaflet with the label STEPS and a picture of stairs on the front. Intrigued, I opened the brochure and read about Central Queensland University's Skills for Tertiary Entry Preparatory Studies (STEPS) course. This was a course for people just like me who couldn't get into any other courses because they didn't finish high school. It was as if someone had read my mind and found the exact course I needed to be able to finally become educated enough to help my kids with their homework! I got chills. I couldn't believe it was just dropped in my letterbox!

I immediately contacted Mum and asked if she would be interested. This was a serious opportunity. I couldn't see myself being able to do it alone and I knew Mum was interested in self-development as well. She agreed. With trepidation, we both applied! We were so excited and nervous but we had each other and, as Mindy had always told us, "What's the worst that can happen?"

There were admission tests and both Mum and I stumbled here. I failed the English test and Mum failed the maths test, both of which were around Year 7 to 8 level. We both had to present for meetings to justify why they should still let us enter the course. We were sitting in the courtyard, waiting for our "show cause" meetings when we made a pact to help each other even if one didn't make it through. If we did make it through, I vowed to help Mum with her maths and she would help me with English.

This was more nerve-wracking than any interview I had ever attended and I vividly remember the depth of that anxiety. This meeting had the potential to confirm what I always thought about myself (that I was stupid) or provide the opportunity to consider an alternative – that I just needed to be more educated! I entered the room shaking and tired from the prior 24 hours of running to the toilet with anxious diarrhoea.

"Tell me, Jodi-Maree, why should we still let you enter the course?"

I repeated the line I gave the lady from TAFE all that time ago: "I will work hard. I will be the best student you ever had."

These people made me feel at ease and by the end I was pretty confident I would get in. Mum and I had each stated our case. We'd both told them how hard we would work to complete the course. We would put extra work into the subjects we were deficient in and help each other to achieve our goals. This time the pleading worked! They let us in! In 1996 we proudly entered the STEPS course as two high school dropouts. Supporting one another, we thrived on our newfound learning capacity and flew through the content.

I had a natural affinity for maths and Mum for English. We didn't just do well, we excelled! Our maths teacher's name was Lois, I will always remember her generosity and loving support. She had a deep belief in what she was doing and went above and beyond for her students. About halfway through the course she sat me down in front of a whiteboard on my own and said, "You know, I think you're capable of doing whatever you want to do, so what do you want to do with your life, Jodi?"

I hadn't really given this any thought; I didn't think there were many possibilities for me. When I was younger, I had volunteered at a veterinary practice and wanted to become a vet but never had the grades or confidence to even consider seriously what else I could do. I had a daydream or two about becoming a doctor and helping people but this felt so out of reach that I never even entertained the thought.

After a couple of minutes of seriously considering my options, I blurted out the most fanciful, "I want to do medicine!" *Why not consider the most difficult and unlikely possibility and go from there?*

Without so much as blinking an eye, Lois flipped over the whiteboard and, with excitement, started writing down the steps I would need to take to achieve this goal. It was a lengthy list and she rambled about each subject as she carefully detailed this pathway on the whiteboard, stating, "You would have to start with adding advanced maths, chemistry, biology. We can get you into bridging versions of all of those subjects so don't worry – that's easy. Then you would have to enrol in biomedical science and apply for the GAMSAT – that's the Graduate Medical School Admissions Test – and that would get you in, providing you did really well in your degree. You would have to get really good grades…"

While she was talking, all I could think of was that this intelligent, educated woman actually thought I could achieve something that seemed so impossible to me. There was no hesitation in her faith in my ability to do this, which made me believe it could be possible. This was the day I learnt how much of a difference one person can make in your life and I vowed to be that person for others wherever I could!

I must have sounded deranged when I proudly announced to anyone who would listen, "I'm going to do medicine." I set about enrolling in all the other subjects I was advised to do. Mum was surprised, but supportive, and continued to complete the STEPS course with me while I did all the additional subjects. It took eight months in total to complete all the necessary prerequisites. Chemistry was difficult, advanced maths was a breeze, and biology was exciting and fun. I got 100 per cent on my final maths test for the STEPS course.

When I saw this result staring back at me, I couldn't believe it. I spent so much of my life telling myself I wasn't smart enough to do something like this. *People like me don't get 100 per cent on a maths test!* I felt a deep sense of pride, and a little bit of hope that I could do this crept in. Once I had all the prerequisites, I sent off my application and nervously awaited the response. I was granted entry into the Bachelor of Biomedical Science at James Cook University in Townsville. I was going to be a uni student. Holding that acceptance letter was so surreal. *This could change our lives.* I hadn't just passed a test; I now had proof that I could rebuild myself from the ground up and overcome that inner voice that held me back for so long. I held my breath. *Maybe I'm not so dumb after all?*

This was a difficult time for me with relationships. I have come to realise that people around you really don't like change. Even when they support you to better yourself, they find it difficult to adapt to a new version of you. Mum was going to drop what she was doing and follow me to Townsville, but I told her I didn't want her to follow me. This had to be very difficult for her – we had started this journey together and I was now separating from her. I needed to know I could survive and thrive without the influence of my parents. This was individuation, and I was desperate to prove myself capable and maybe even intelligent. The little voice in my head that told me *Don't be so stupid, you can't do this, you're not smart enough* was louder than ever and I was fighting this self-doubt every day. It was exhausting. I had an inner strength that came from being a mum to two beautiful children. I couldn't let them down, I had to become a better version of myself, I had to create a better future for them!

I insisted on my new path despite the resistance and moved to Townsville at the end of 1996. Mum was really upset and we didn't talk for a while. She later told me she felt rejected and, while that wasn't my intention, I recognise how hard this must have been for her. She moved interstate to live so we only spoke over the phone for a while. The kids seemed to have no problem adapting to their new environment. Excited but terrified of failure, I started life as a first-year university student, this time without any ties to my parents.

As adult children, we often neglect to consider the impact we have on our parents as human beings. It took some time for me to change my perception and see Mum and Dad as fallible, humans who made mistakes just like the rest of us. I had unfair and unreasonable expectations of Mum at this time, still harbouring some unresolved anger from my childhood and her inability to keep me safe. On reflection, the cycle of abuse is complicated; Mum never really knew anything other than mistreatment her whole life. This really saddens me now. I did a lot of work in my later life to show her what an unconditional, safe relationship looks like. I can only hope this gave her some degree of restoration.

UNLEARNING STUPID

Once there was a little girl, her name was Jo
She often spent her days feeling so very low
She was told she would never make it in life
She always found herself in some kind of strife
Believing every harsh word that had ever been said
The words stupid and subordinate swirled around in her head
When she had children of her own, she worried so much
How could she help them with school when she was so out of touch?
With a newfound confidence and belief in herself
Jo went back to school, adding textbooks to her shelf
She finished one degree then started one more
Until she finally proved she wasn't stupid, for sure
The battle was internal, how hard she had fought
Never again would she give those harsh words a second thought

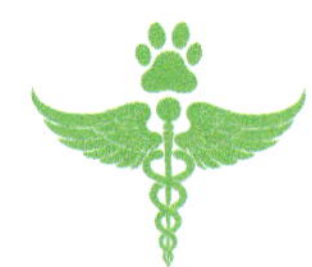

It was orientation, or O week, and I was in awe of the university campus and surrounded by the buzz of intelligent people. It felt like I was the only clown in the circus and at some point people would realise I was in the wrong place! There were exciting "shows" in the science lab – stalls with senior students recommending their courses and faculties. It was like going to the local agricultural show, only better because I felt like I was a part of something bigger than myself.

This was also North Queensland and we had a weather event closing in. Sometime in O week, Tropical Cyclone Justin made its presence known. I was on an orientation tour with other students when an announcement was made that local schools and daycare centres would be closing due to the cyclone. I had struck up a conversation with a young, intelligent, 17-year-old boy who was also doing biomedical science, Graeme Kay. At the time, he was shocked when I announced I would have to go to pick up my children from daycare.

"You're a mum?" He sounded surprised. I didn't have too much time to elaborate so I told him how important my two beautiful kids were to me and headed off to pick them up. The next time I saw Graeme he was asking for a lift to class and, from then on, we were inseparable! He became part of the family, sitting in between the kids on rides to uni, and we discussed every difficult assignment or concept at length. He was an intellectual and we spent hours discussing complex concepts and the problems of the world! I loved those conversations; they kept me engaged in the course content. I didn't know it at the time but this was the start of a lifetime friendship with a very special human being.

We connected with a group of people who were all interested in getting into medicine and met once a week to talk about various topics. We mused and complained about the difference in workload for biomedical science students, with the 27 hours a week contact time blitzing some of the other disciplines. Some of the subjects were easier than others for my deficient brain and chemistry was my nemesis. Although I had completed the basic chemistry prerequisites, I just didn't understand it very well. This was extremely frustrating and became both a source of tension and a challenge to overcome. Both Mum and Dad had taught me to persist when things were tough and this would serve me well at university.

Lois's whiteboard picture was flashing in my head with every assessment, along with her words: *You will have to get really good grades.* The internal pressure to be both a good mum and achieve academically weighed heavily on me; finding the balance was my daily challenge. Angelina had to go into daycare and Eliot would sometimes have to go to after- or before-school care for me to complete my degree. I was adamant the kids were not in daycare more than they had to be, so I took classes at night. This meant I could be at home during the day while they were awake and so I could be the one to pick them up and drop them off as often as possible.

I also had a self-imposed rule that I would only study once they had gone to bed so that our time together as a family was focused on them. This was the beginning of many years of self-imposed sleep deprivation. I learnt how to play their video games so we could play together and I could help them if they got stuck, and we would run to the fence and back in the rain for fun. I felt a bit of maternal guilt going to university and putting them in daycare. I didn't want my study to have a negative impact on them so I minimised it wherever I could. After all, they were the whole reason I was doing this! The people around me were all made acutely aware that my children came first. "If you hurt my kids, I *will* kill you!" became a running joke within the group, but I was only half joking!

I wanted to be sure anyone around me knew that the kids were my absolute priority.

With every successful assessment, every good grade, my confidence grew. In first year, I sat the undergraduate medical admissions test (UMAT) in an attempt to fast-track my entry into medicine, but I got a dismal result so had to continue in the biomedical science degree. I had a renewed sense of how hard I would have to work to get into medicine, so I set about working harder and fighting for every grade, every mark. In second year, I won the university prize for Academic Excellence in Biochemistry. You would think that meant I loved the subject, but that wasn't the case. This happened because I found chemistry in general so arduous! There were many nights spent agonising over assessments and trying to understand concepts. Sometimes it was so difficult I would cry in frustration. This would challenge me, sometimes pushing my brain and nervous system to their limits.

Mum had moved back to Mackay and her support was also much appreciated. The second year of any degree is difficult because you can't see the light at the end of the tunnel. The subject material and workload intensify, and assessments continue to pile up seemingly without relief. Towards the end of second year, I started to see the light. It became easier to knuckle down and get the work done, and all the hard work in the earlier parts of the course set a good foundation for doing well. That year, Graeme and I volunteered at a local biotechnology company called TropBio to improve our chances of getting into medicine. Being a university student and now working at TropBio, I felt a deep sense of purpose. I was excited about what the future would bring, and each day brought new facts and learning that stimulated my brain. I was a sponge, soaking up all the goodness, leaving not a morsel of the learning untouched.

Despite the joy of being at university, the realities of raising a family and studying were never far from the surface. I was constantly trying to balance finances, the need to be there for the kids and the need to perform at university. This would be the beginning of trying to fit life in between.

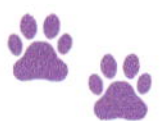

Somewhere in this year, during one of our many six-hour practical's at the biochemistry lab, we were sitting outside, waiting for a reaction in our experiment to complete, when we saw something funny. A young male student was walking across the vast green area in front of us under the canopy of many large trees, including some gum trees. Graeme and I were watching him as he suddenly flicked his hands around his head as if swooshing away an insect of some sort. We both noticed it and had a little giggle but thought no more of it until the next person walked through the same path across the grass and under the trees, this time getting quite animated, not only swooshing at their head but also smacking themselves on the arms and legs. By now we were in fits of laughter and had realised there must have been some bees swarming around these people as they walked through.

In between our fits of laughter, another lady walked past the same spot. Predictably she started swooshing at her head and arms just like the others, quickly turning her leisurely walk into a bee ballet that would rival any Swan Lake performance. She frantically started flicking up her skirt, twisting her body into unnatural positions and tossing her bags at the invisible culprits. Tears of laughter ensued. It was a battle between dignity and survival and, so far, it was bees – three, students – nil. We could no longer watch the carnage. Our sense of responsibility had finally kicked in and we let someone know that there must be some bees over there, so no-one else would have to suffer the same fate. Still retelling and laughing about our little adventure, we went back to complete our six-hour practical, having filled in a suitable amount of time with the frivolity. Moments like these were common during my time at university and I still look back on them fondly.

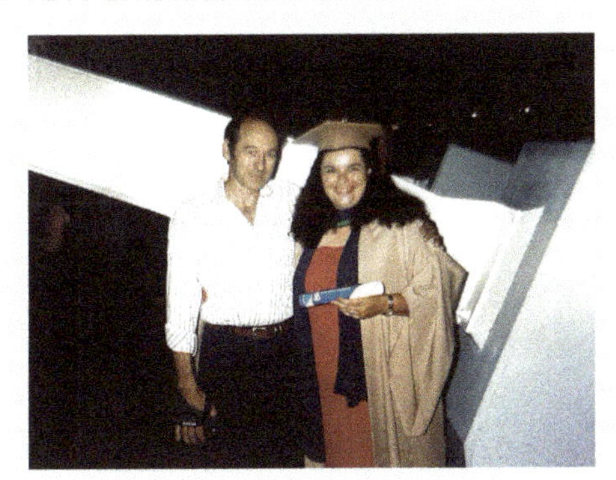

Dad at my graduation from biomedical science

In third year, I won the same biochemistry prize as well as the Ashdown Medal for Clinical Microbiology and the Patterson Medal for Immunology. Academic performance was essential if I was going to achieve the desired result. I was mostly competing with myself but a friend and fellow future doctor, Amy (we called her big A), was a constant source of inspiration to me and this pushed both of us to do better. Between us, we topped our graduating year and won most of the prizes on offer. I had done it! I had graduated from biomedical science with university medals and awards, but I still had that nagging voice in my head: *You're so stupid!*

My graduation from James Cook University occurred after we moved out of our house, so we were temporarily staying in a little caravan. My father only came to the ceremony because he was pressured by family to attend, and he and Nang arrived at the caravan I was staying in. I had purchased a pack of cards to give to my friends to congratulate them on their amazing achievement.

"Do you have any spare cards?" Dad asked.

"Yes," I said, handing him one.

"Bend over for a sec."

I complied and he leaned on my back as he wrote a message on one of the cards, put the card in the envelope and handed it to me before walking out to attend the ceremony. I opened the card and read his message: "Jodi – that's one down and two to go!"

I started to sob. *It isn't enough! He's still not proud of me.* I understood what he was saying in the card – that I now had to finish the Bachelor of Medicine, Bachelor of Surgery double degree before he would be satisfied. I was devastated. His disrespect and flippant disregard for the last three years of work and sacrifice had really upset me, but that quickly turned to anger. I attended the ceremony, smiling on the outside, but internally I was deflated and deeply demoralised. I congratulated my friends and collected my degree, but a fire had been lit in my soul. *I'll show you! I* will *become a doctor then you will finally know how wrong you were about me!*

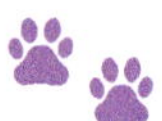

I had completed the GAMSAT before final exams and my score was actually pretty good. This test was very different from the undergraduate one – the questions were more logical and scientific, and the content less obscure. I'd been offered an interview but had very limited funds. Unfortunately, I had to get some financial assistance to afford to go as I just had no way of getting to this interview otherwise. I was so grateful that I vowed to repay this small kindness one day. Dad conditioned me to believe relationships are transactional. You had to get something in return if you did something for someone and vice versa. He did this in many ways but one of the ways I remember was when he would offer to do something like take you to the movies. You would have to iron his shirt, massage or clean his back, or do some other task before you earnt this reward. I always felt like I had to pay back any kindness, gesture, help or support. This has often made me feel like I'm only of value to people if I'm giving them something or doing something for them. While no-one once asked for anything in return, because of my conditioning, I would always find a way to return any kindness afforded me sometime in the future.

I was overweight, so it was hard to find something nice enough for such an important interview, but I finally found a blue, two-piece, professional-looking suit. The interview was intimidating, with a panel of people firing questions at me. I was fine until they asked me who I would choose if one of my children was sick and I also had a sick patient to tend to. Even at the time, I found this to be an odd question as it's not one they would be able to ask everyone. I responded the only way I knew how, with honesty. I would always choose my children, and I would call in sick. They enquired further, doubling down on their focus on family versus professional responsibility, asking, "What if there was no-one to cover your shift?" I didn't know how to answer this so I just reiterated that my family would always come first and there were systems in place to allow for this.

I guess dedication to family is what they wanted to hear as I apparently did very well on this interview. However, I wasn't offered a place in the first round of offers and, after graduating, just wanted to kick back and relax. I reasoned that, like my friend Graeme, I may need to do an honours year to get into medicine anyway. I had already discussed my honours project and sorted out who would be my supervisor. The only thing left to do was to put in the application. Now that I knew I wasn't getting into medicine, this would be my next focus.

While getting ready to visit family and friends in Mackay, I was in the kitchen when the phone rang. I answered the phone, "Hello?"

On the other end of the line was a man who introduced himself as a member of the medical admissions team and said that someone had pulled out and my name was next on the list. He said there was a position in the University of Melbourne's Bachelor of Medicine, Bachelor of Surgery program. "That's if you still want it."

I had to control my urge to scream down the phone and instead, relatively excitedly, said, "Yes, yes, of course I still want it!"

He proceeded to tell me that I would receive the formal offer in the mail in the next week and, as it was a graduate program, I would start halfway through the year. I got off the phone, and then the squealing began… I think they could hear me all the way from Melbourne!

"I got in! I got in!"

Excitement filled the house, and soon the kids were also jumping and squealing. The trip down to see the family now had a completely different tone. I waited until we got there and the first person I shared the news with was my mum. She was so excited for me and jumped up and down with me, then got a bit sad that I would have to move away again. My dad was predictably unfazed. I think he said something like, "Oh, that's good."

Then I shared with everyone I knew. While most people were happy for me, some gave a completely different, unusual and unexpected response. Some seemed to think I was being selfish or irresponsible doing this to my children again after having just spent three years in relative poverty. I was dumbfounded by this response.

My excitement had turned to concern. *Is this going to be unfair to the kids? Is this the wrong thing to do? Am I really just being selfish? Surely, I'm doing what's best for my family?* After some discussion and calming down a little, I was convinced I was doing the right thing for my little family by creating a secure future for them, and they would understand in the long run. However, it had been a difficult few years financially. I needed to be responsible and minimise the impact this decision would have on my family, so I decided I would also get some part-time work. After contemplating this carefully, I started to feel that perhaps some people found it challenging to see me achieving. In my view, I was never expected to become anything significant so perhaps this was a difficult transition for others. I didn't realise it then, but I was doing what very few people even attempt, rebuilding my life while trying to raise a family.

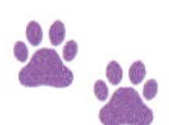

We stayed with Dad and Nang, helping them renovate their house in Mackay, while we waited for the mid-year start. One of the advantages of your best friend marrying your father is that we always got along very well. Being at Dad and Nang's house worked well as I could put our belongings in storage and stay closer to family before moving away. I spent as much time as I could with the kids, doing whatever fun things we could afford. Finally a little house in a suburb near Melbourne became available. I felt accomplished, like I had kept the promise I made when they were babies to create a better future for them. I felt like this would be a new and better path for both of the children, one that would create generational healing and lasting security.

I wanted to find a nice place, outside the city and all its potential negative influences, where the kids would be safe growing up. Sunbury was just far enough away and just close enough for public transport to uni. The University of Melbourne was an exciting, buzzing environment and some of its buildings were spectacular. It took an hour and 20 minutes each way for me to commute on public transport but I enjoyed the trip and it would give me the opportunity to do some uni work on the train to avoid cutting into the time I had with the kids.

In our orientation we were all corralled into a large lecture theatre for an "inspirational" talk about what lay ahead for us as medical students. One of the many speakers that day was a very formal-looking gentleman, with a very long title and many, many letters after his name. He stood up in front of us and launched into a speech that, I felt, dripped in privilege. If I thought I was a fish out of water in biomedical science, I was a goldfish in a sea of sharks in medicine! He talked about how we were the "top two per cent of students in Australia" – *I know he doesn't mean me* – how 30 per cent of us wouldn't make it through the course – *Will this be me?* – and 50 per cent of those left would become general practitioners. *Is that a bad thing?*

I felt very out of place. I got into this profession to help people, because I genuinely cared about people, and this speech made me feel incredibly inadequate. I wondered how many of the people in this audience felt the same way I did. Then it occurred to me that maybe, in this elite environment, I was in the minority. Not many people around me came from social disadvantage and how many of them had children?

How many had to work to make ends meet? How many had a trauma background, having experienced coercive control? Was there anyone there like me? Others around me seemed inspired by this speech but I felt more terrified than ever and immediately felt isolated and exposed. *Surely someone will discover that I'm not that smart. Someone will realise I don't belong here. Then all this work will have been for nothing. All I will have done is disadvantage my beautiful children, just like the naysayers had said. So much for creating a better future! What have I done?*

While the university was amazing, with world-class teaching and an incredible support program, my conditioning was kicking in and I was overwhelmed by my inadequacies again. I was deeply concerned that I'd made a mistake. I just had to stay positive as I uprooted my whole family to accept this opportunity. There had been so many sacrifices to get to this point. If this didn't work out, it would all be on me! The pressure was enormous – I had to make this work! I set about finding some friends who were mature age or that I had something in common with. I was grateful to find some good friends and this made me feel a bit less isolated. However, I missed my biomedical science friends, particularly Graeme. He stayed on for an honour's year and while we still kept in touch, it wasn't the same. This period was very lonely. I wouldn't say the work was any more difficult than biomed. It just went at a faster pace, and the pass mark was set higher so it was much harder to stand out or do well. I guess you don't want a doctor who knows less than 70 per cent of the material!

I got through the first year and did relatively well, not having to be too concerned with the "pass" mark as my grades were consistently higher than that. I was managing to find time to be with the kids by studying after they went to bed, and I was still working. One of the benefits of university is all the holidays you get to spend with your family. The commute was killing me but I did manage to get some work done on the train. I had settled into the course by second semester, second year and I was spending so much time privately tutoring that there wasn't really any time to socialise. I didn't have a lot of friends and never stayed back to participate in social events as I much preferred to spend that time at home with my family. I was also nervous about being at home alone overnight in Sunbury when my husband was at work, so whenever this occurred it impacted on my sleep. *I just have to get over it!* I worked very hard to manage anxiety related to my trauma history, and eventually came to a place where I could sleep soundly and not have to barricade the door or check for safety, disrupting my sleep. I often feel guilty when I remember this time, worrying about any potential impact my anxieties may have had on the kids.

The second half of the course would be spent on rotations through different specialties in medicine. Rotations were six-month periods spent in different locations, exploring various specialties and subspecialties. This meant potentially moving every six months or spending six months at a time away from my family. To me it was obvious that this course wasn't designed for families! Luckily for us they had developed a Rural Clinical School, which provided an alternative option. This was in a lovely little rural Victorian town and it meant I wouldn't have to move the family around every six months for my course. Naturally, I decided this was the best option for our little family. I remember this as a particularly happy time.

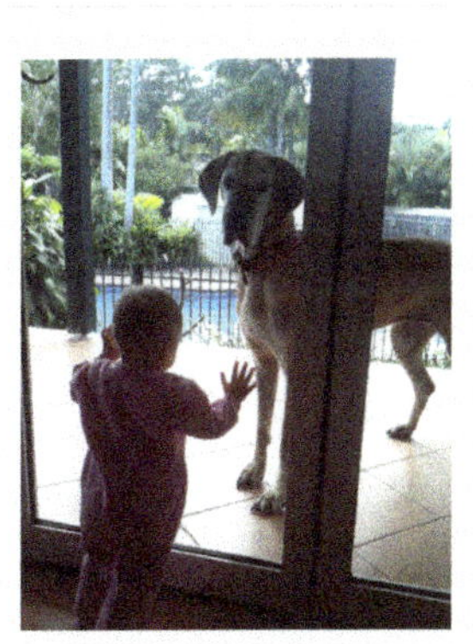

Honey the beautiful Great Dane

The Rural Clinical School was a supportive and friendly environment. We lived on a rural property with an apple orchard out the back and room for animals. Because of my affinity with the breed, we got a beautiful Great Dane we called Honey (just like my childhood pet)

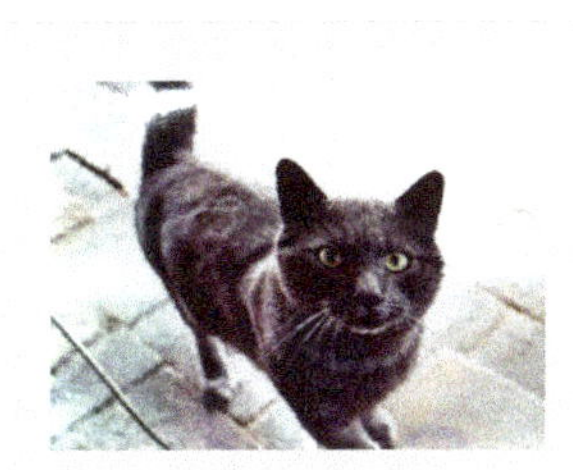

Mars the incredible cat

and a cat called Mars. We were in our element – a lovely rural property with family pets! We also had another dog for a while, but we eventually found a farm home for her. The dogs both had puppies and the kids got to experience what it was like to care for these little babies. There was never much money while I was a full-time student, but we had a car, a roof over our heads, family pets and the kids had everything they needed so we were doing okay.

Studying medicine was very humbling. There were so many things that could go wrong with the human body and so many ways we, as doctors, could help or hurt depending on our level of knowledge and skill. Psychiatry was a particularly interesting rotation for me, and I learnt a lot about myself and my family throughout this unit. I was able to make sense of my childhood, and better understand Mum and Dad's upbringings and how they shaped them as parents. I had spent countless hours doing internal work to process the childhood trauma I experienced.

Medicine was also humbling academically; I had fallen from the top of the class to the middle, with so many amazingly intelligent people well above me. While I found some very good friends, I also felt quite lonely. It was isolating being surrounded by young, privileged people, many of whom had parents who paid their way. I often had difficulty communicating with them as they talked about their new designer clothes, or the dilemma of which new technology or gadget to buy next, while I considered which bill to pay this week, how to afford the new school shoes required, or how to buy the best new game or toy for the kids. Some of the other students seemed to find it difficult to understand why I would skip a class to be at home with the kids if they were sick, go to their school fair, or choose the kids' awards ceremony over attending the weekly student get-together. They were wonderful, intelligent people who would make fantastic doctors, but we came from completely different worlds and it was frequently, painfully obvious that I didn't fit in. Having said that, I don't think I ever fit in anywhere.

The Rural Clinical School was a wonderful time in the medicine journey for me and I believe it was enjoyable for the kids too. I always had the ethos that we were a package deal as a family so if the kids couldn't come to an event I wouldn't attend either. We joined the local badminton club and a few of us students started to volunteer at the local community centre, offering free community talks about contraception, teen pregnancy and other women's health issues.

In my Obstetrics and Gynaecology (O&G) rotation I developed a deep interest in women's health and discovered my calling was O&G.

In final year, so close to the finish line, my car died. I had no capacity to fix it and if I couldn't find a way to replace it, I would have to defer. This would have been devastating so close to the finish line. I approached the dean of the Rural Clinical School and she advised there was an emergency bursary I could apply for. I applied and got a $3,000 bursary, and I went down to the auctions to buy a car. I purchased a little Mitsubishi Magna wagon, which got me through to the end of the degree. I would have done almost anything to get to the finish line after spending eight years of my life getting to that point. It's like the accumulation of lactic acid in a marathon – you just have to push through!

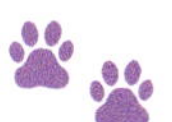

In my graduating year I won the Simon Furphy Prize for contribution to the local community and passed my final exams. Believe me when I say final exams in medicine felt like a whole other world of stress and anxiety. We were sequestered in a locked room and sent out one at a time to do each of the stations. The stations could be anything from the entire medical degree and would include history, physical examination, diagnostics and management plans. If you failed this exam, this year, you didn't graduate with everyone else. My anxiety was at an all-time high and I was physically ill before this pressure cooker of an exam. We were all so relieved to have gotten through it and even more relieved to have passed! I wasn't coming out the other side of this degree the same person as I went in. So much had changed, I had processed and worked through many of my fears, anxieties and inadequacies.

I jokingly told my father he would be disowned if he didn't come to my graduation. I offered to help pay for him to come, but he reassured me he would be there, "Come hell or high water."

I had even sent out an invitation to make sure he knew he was invited. The actual ceremony had a limit to the number of people who could attend so only family could actually be inside for the ceremony. There was one other person I really wanted there; my beautiful friend, Graeme Kay. He turned up for me as he always had, waiting for me outside the hall. Graeme was now a medical student himself at the University of Queensland and we had come a long way together, so he knew better than most how important this day was.

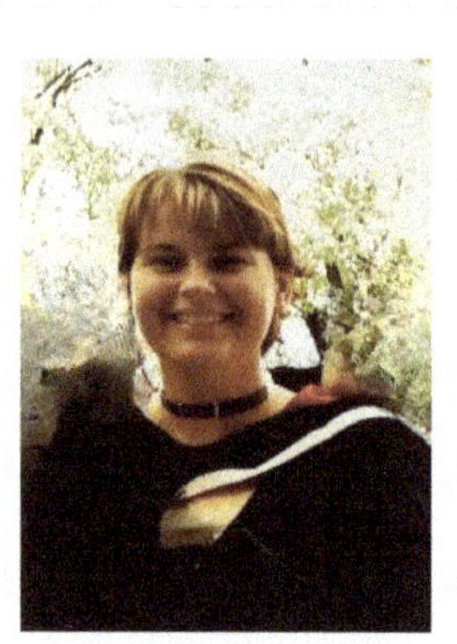

Graduation from Medicine

Graduation was regal with all the pomp and ceremony you could imagine. I was in my beautiful gown and looking forward to the after-party. My lovely little family was there looking up at me and Graeme was waiting for me outside. When they called my name, all the negative adjectives that had been used to describe me throughout my life, *stupid, idiot, subordinate*, and all the feelings of inadequacy flashed before me as I walked up to the podium. I could hear the Whitney Houston song *One Moment in Time* playing in my head. This was my one moment. I was more than I ever thought I could be. Tears welled in my eyes as I proudly shook the hand of the presenter. I felt that little voice that used to say *You can't, you're too stupid* get crushed under the weight of this achievement. I never heard that voice again. It disappeared that day and never returned!

I went home to an after-party filled with family and friends who were excited, celebrating the achievement of a lifetime with me. The only person missing was my dad. I tried to call him, but he wasn't answering and it became clear that he wasn't coming. He wasn't even going to congratulate me. After trying a few times to reach him, I quietly went inside the house and cried. Mum came in to console me and couldn't believe he didn't show up on such an important occasion. I wasn't going to let his behaviour ruin my night the way it had ruined my other graduation, so I allowed myself a few minutes to mourn and then let go of the years of approval seeking, gathering myself together to rejoin the party. I knew that he would never be proud of me no matter what I achieved, and he would never admit that he was wrong. I also knew beyond a shadow of a doubt that this was his problem, not mine! *I am enough, I am intelligent and I am no-one's fool.*

I rejoined the party and celebrated like there was no tomorrow. I stood up and gave my husband his honorary medical degree, publicly acknowledging him for his flexibility and undying support, recognising all the sacrifices I felt he had to make to get us here, and thanked my beautiful children for their patience and encouragement. The kids were always my biggest cheer squad, and their support and love meant a lot to me! This journey had started with a desire to help them with their homework and, if not for them, I don't think I would have ever had the strength to do something so challenging. I also thanked my family and friends for their ongoing support, and for turning up for me both physically and psychologically on such an important day. I had done it! It was over! I had defeated my inner demons. I applied for an internship in a regional centre and set about getting ready for this exciting time. Time to enjoy being an intern, finally have an income and reap the rewards of the past eight years of sacrifice.

LOVE

They told me what love is, but I think I misunderstood
I thought love meant caring for others and giving everything I could
They told me what love is, but I think I may have misheard
In the name of love I gave all I had, remaining undeterred
They told me what love is, but I might have got it wrong
I gave all my love to others, thinking it would make me strong
They told me what love is, and I think I made a mistake
Giving all I had to others, there was nothing left but heartache
I thought I knew what love is, but clearly it was untrue
In only ever loving others what gets lost is you

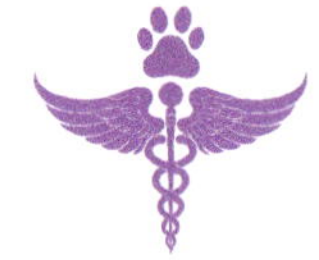

To say that I loved being a doctor would be an understatement. It was the most privileged position to be in and I had achieved this position through blood, sweat, tears and sacrifice. As a doctor you get to see people at their most vulnerable, and how you treat and care for them makes a difference, sometimes to their emotional wellbeing but sometimes to their survival.

There is a hierarchy in medicine and the intern is at the bottom. The next level up is an RMO (resident medical officer), registrar (junior and then senior trainee), a fellow (advanced trainee/subspecialist trainee) and then a consultant (the head honcho). As rewarding as it was, the job was a real challenge! I would sometimes come face to face with some complex personalities. At times, I perceived challenging behaviours in the senior clinicians and the odd entitled, overinflated, egotistical junior doctor, and even the public health system in general – similar to what I experienced with my dad.

Don't get me wrong. Most of my colleagues were beautiful, compassionate people who were there for the same reason as me, to genuinely help people, but there were also a few who seemed to have way too much power or be really hard to deal with at times. Intern year was an assault on all the senses – from being covered in bodily fluids with smells so foreign you can't describe, seeing some of the horrible things people do to one another, hearing the screams and cries of a wailing mother in labour, experiencing the feel of crackling burnt skin, and the bad taste you get in your mouth when you shovel the very old, very cold dinner in before you see the next patient.

I learnt very quickly there's great responsibility in medicine, and you need to respect it and be humble. I wasn't used to working full-time as a doctor, but I was keen to do the job well and I was rostered on for the weekend. In the final hours of what felt like a long, arduous weekend shift, just before handover I realised that I had made a very small but potentially serious mistake. In medical school it was drummed into us that mistakes as an intern can cost lives, so I was extremely cautious and diligent. I checked everything twice but when you're fatigued, that level of diligence just isn't enough! I had charted one of my patients a bag of fluids with potassium replacement as their potassium was a bit low.

This was a very regular occurrence on the wards. However, instead of giving it to the appropriate patient, I had charted it for someone else with a similar name and only realised my error while I was doing handover. I immediately called my registrar (the doctor on shift above me in authority) and admitted my mistake, asked the nurse to take down the fluids and notified each of the patients. The patients were very understanding, and the registrar was very supportive, basically agreeing with my plan, adding that I would also have to follow protocol, tell the consultant and file an incident report.

I didn't care about getting in trouble or filing a report but I was terrified that the person who wrongly received the potassium may have some sort of cardiac event as a result of my error. Thankfully, their bloods came back confirming their potassium was still in the normal range. The other patient had their bag of potassium as their levels were still low. Disaster averted, but lesson learnt! If I was going to get through and be good at this job I needed to be more vigilant, especially when fatigued.

Over the course of the intern year, I learnt that at around 13 consecutive hours of work, you hit a wall and must stop to be safe. However, after that you can just keep going until you got to go home. Sometimes you would voluntarily stay behind to help a colleague or because there was an interesting case to manage. Compared to stories about the long shifts of our predecessors, interns now seemed well protected in terms of safe work hours. I learnt that the other doctors seemed to palm off the boring and more unpleasant (code for something stuck in a patient's nether region somewhere) cases to the intern. To me it also seemed that if you were right about something obscure or serious as a junior doctor, you were unlikely to be believed, but a senior doctor was much more likely to be believed if they said the same thing. Like many professions, credibility came with experience.

In my intern year I had an amazing friend who made life fun and interesting. Kareem was charming, witty, funny and very intelligent. He made intern year fun! We did a general medical rotation together and we would go on ward rounds together to support each other, which was deemed a little strange by others but made our day easier. On these ward rounds he would randomly walk behind me while a rather serious dissertation was occurring, with the expectation that our full attention be on the super important consultant while they spoke in case some hidden gem of a tip would fall from their golden lips. Kareem would wait for the perfect moment to whisper a completely random, anatomically inappropriate word (usually related to genitalia) in an attempt to break my resolute focus on the consultant. This irreverence made every day with Kareem a pleasure and it taught me you need to keep both a sense of humour and a straight face to survive in this job.

On one of these amazing ward rounds, and after surviving several of Kareem's hilarious attempts to derail me, I began presenting my patient who had ovarian cancer and had been complaining of abdominal pain. I didn't get past her presenting issue (abdominal pain) before the normally serious and seemingly frightening consultant we affectionately referred to as "Aunty Sage", who was known for her brilliance in bedside diagnostics, piped up.

She blurted out, "No shit, Sherlock. She has ovarian cancer."

She was still chuckling under her breath while the patient and other junior doctors were in hysterics at my blindingly obvious statement. I immediately saw the funny side and, while another person may have been offended, this doctor made me feel at ease. It was in this moment that I realised this consultant was just like me. She wasn't scary at all. She was just a doctor doing her job and she needed to find light in her day, just like we did. I believe she would probably be horrified to know this changed how I saw consultants forever.

While I always had professional respect for them, I also demanded respect as a fellow human being. While we were improving as a profession, it still seemed common for consultants to humiliate or berate junior doctors on ward rounds, an outdated and unhealthy way to learn. After experiencing Aunty Sage and the fear her presence seemed to strike into the hearts of junior doctors, I decided I would no longer accept that for myself as I was also a human doing the best I could. This would get me in trouble from time to time but for the most part consultants seemed to respect me when I stood up for myself, much like Dad had all those years ago. This acceptance of consultants as fellow human beings first, and respected colleagues second, made it easier for me to get along with some very difficult people in medicine. This would be a distinct advantage later in my career.

The misconceptions around junior doctor salaries were rife. Nursing staff would often say things like, "That's why you get paid the big bucks," without knowing that many nursing staff got paid higher hourly rates. We had no unions, so the nurses had better working conditions and often they seemed more likely to be supported by their colleagues if something went wrong. As a junior doctor, the nursing staff were my best friends!

Without them I would have struggled to get through. They often knew the nuances of each of the consultants and would remind you if you had forgotten to do something the consultant would want you to have finished by the time they got to the ward. They also frequently picked up any minor medication charting errors, putting them on the board, often with a little note that said something like "Just saved your ass."

The nursing staff were a ray of sunshine in even the darkest of times. I often felt like I had more in common with the nurses or midwives than I did with my medical colleagues.

One of the advantages of this year was that, as a family, we would finally have money coming in! At the end of my first fortnight as an intern, I eagerly awaited the deposit of my first pay as a doctor into my bank account. I was kind of desperate for money by this stage as my Centrelink payments had ended, and all the student financial supports had well and truly dried up. I went into the office the next day to see the Junior Medical Officer (JMO) manager only to find that I had forgotten to put in my timesheet! I was so excited and nervous about my first two weeks as a doctor that I simply forgot about getting paid. Luckily, my stint as the intern cohort's comic relief didn't last too long. There was a rush put on the payment for me and it was in the bank within 24 hours… I never forgot to put in a payslip again in my intern year.

This newfound wealth would be used to move into a new, more comfortable rental closer to the hospital, which I would set about filling with fun stuff like a pool table, dart board, games room and musical instruments for the kids. I would invite every new rotation of interns to the house for dinner, to welcome them to our little rural hospital, and the kids would play them music.

I felt so incredibly proud to be providing for the family, but, in reality, a lot of these things were going on my credit card. I reasoned that I would have the income to pay them off. This house was affectionately referred to as "the house of fun" and boy did we have some fun here. We started to do things we could never afford before, like going out to dinner and special events. I desperately wanted to make up for the years the family had spent sacrificing for me to finish my degree. I wanted to make our lives and their childhood as stable, easy and fun as I could.

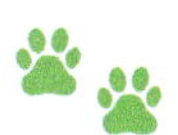

My interest in O&G continued in my intern year, but the prospect of specialising in this field was getting further out of my grasp. To do this specialty I would have to apply for, and gain entry to, the College of Obstetricians and Gynaecologists training program, which would involve rotating placements every six months for the next six years. The family had already given up so much for my training. I felt like getting into O&G training would be truly selfish given the sacrifices they had already made. With my focus on making the family happy, I looked at places to live where they could be happy and I could get a job.

I discovered that I could become a general practitioner (GP) and do O&G as a GP without having to move the family around for my training. I found a suitable place I thought the family would love on the coast, with beaches and a good climate, secured a job for myself and set about moving. Arriving on December 24, to a house I agreed to solely from an internet viewing in the searing heat, this would become affectionately known as "home crap home"!

This house looked ideal on the internet. It was on several acres of land, we could have pets for the kids, and I wanted to get a horse again so I could ride in my "spare" time. This little property had no cupboards, no window coverings and no heating or cooling. The garage had been struck by lightning and the electricity in there wasn't functional or safe, and the house had absolutely no character. The grass was about waist height for me, so the entire property was completely unsafe for Mars and Honey, let alone the children. It was Christmas Eve so none of this was going to be addressed anytime soon. All we could do was laugh about it and make do with what we had. At least there were some good beaches for the kids, better than sweltering in the Besser block cooker of a house. It quickly became clear that the online listing had been a triumph in optimism - a "special" kind of unintended Christmas gift.

My RMO year was difficult, with rotations in paediatrics, as well as general surgery and medicine, both of which I disliked. However, I absolutely loved teaching, didn't mind paediatrics, and my great love,

O&G, was still my calling. Spare time became laughable for me due to all the overtime. I was now proud to be the typical hard-working junior doctor. The Mitsubishi Magna that got me through the final year of medicine finally died so I took out a small loan to buy a second-hand, reliable Toyota Camry with low kilometres. Close to the end of my RMO year I secured a position in the department of O&G as a second-year RMO with the hopes it would turn into an unaccredited registrar position, and I could complete my GP diploma in O&G.

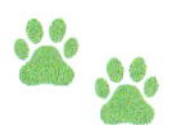

In 2006, I had the great privilege of attending my friend Graeme's graduation from medicine at the University of Queensland. What an amazing achievement and I just knew that he was going to make an incredible doctor. We had now both completed something we set out to do together so many years earlier and I was so proud of him!

We moved into a new rental property closer to the hospital in anticipation of the potential for longer hours and on-call shifts that would come with any future registrar role. This house was a huge overcompensation for the past 12 months spent in the misery of home crap home. The "mansion" had three levels, a swimming pool, a kids' retreat, a huge yard for the animals, and all the bells and whistles of luxury. It was significantly more expensive, but I could afford it as I would be on a registrar's salary. The mansion was decked out with all the fun you could imagine. The house was filled with the kind of things kids dream about – games, gear, music and room to play. I could afford to enrol the kids in whatever extracurricular activities they wanted and keep up with anything their friends may have enjoyed. It felt like proof the years of sacrifice had finally paid off.

The RMO year in O&G was fantastic! I absolutely loved this job. It was hard work but an incredibly privileged time to be involved in a woman's life. Anything could go wrong at any time, which made the job very exciting as no two shifts were ever the same. I also loved the staff in this little unit. The midwives were an incredible source of support to me as a junior doctor and they were becoming dear friends. I was aware that doing your job well could save a life and that was pretty special. Doing your job poorly could also end a life and the gravity of that stayed with me throughout my working life.

Death is part of the cycle of life and, as a junior medical officer, certifying death is also part of the job. Thankfully, I never experienced a maternal death in my working life but I had the misfortune of experiencing many foetal deaths in utero (death during pregnancy, after 20 weeks and before birth) and a few neonatal deaths (death following a live birth and up to 28 days after birth) as well. This is just part of the job but there's something so tragic about the loss of such a young life and it always hit me hard.

I vividly remember the first patient whose death I had to certify. It was in my intern year. I was very inexperienced professionally and had absolutely no life experience with human death apart from my high school boyfriend's best mate. This patient had a progressively degenerative condition that had gradually caused their deterioration. Our team was taking care of her so I had gotten to know the family and the patient well. She was a very sick woman but always found time to be polite and grateful to every member of her treating team. One morning, after our rounds on the ward, a nurse quietly approached me and pulled me aside.

"Bed 4 has passed and I need you to examine her and document her death."

The nurse was so gentle, respectful and kind. I went through in my head what I needed to do to certify death and headed to her room to examine her. I was a little nervous, having never done this before, but the nurse was experienced and so supportive. She stayed with me every step of the way.

There were familiar family members quietly grieving in the room as I went about my formal examination. I made sure that at each step I checked with the family and answered any questions they had. I started the examination by stating, "Just confirming this is Mrs Smith."

The nurse responded, "Yes, Mrs Smith." We went on to confirm her date of birth and hospital identification number. I listened for heart sounds, felt and listened for breathing, checked that she was non-responsive to pain stimuli, and that her pupils were fixed and not reactive to light.

There were no signs of life and I communicated this to the family, "I'm so sorry but I can confirm Mrs Smith has passed away."

The family were all prepared for this eventuality but still actively grieved as I left the room. I went into the office where the interns did their paperwork, shed a little tear, and pulled myself together to complete the death certificate and document the examination I had just completed. The gravity of this experience weighed on me heavily for the rest of the day and I had a quick, private cry when I got home, paying my respects to this woman and her family the only way I knew how. This was my first encounter with death in medicine but it definitely wouldn't be my last. Death in obstetrics and gynaecology always felt like a more harrowing experience.

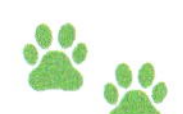

I went on to become an O&G registrar and commenced my diploma in obstetrics and gynaecology. I sat the exam and did well, commencing in general practice as originally intended. I had the absolute pleasure of working with some amazing human beings, one of whom was my friend, Nele. Nele was a registrar from Germany. She was friendly, kind, incredibly skilled and a pleasure to work with. We worked and played together during her six-month rotation, with her spending lovely time getting to know me and my family. Horse riding and social dinners were also on the menu. She was an amazing source of inspiration for me and we remain friends to this day.

One of the harder parts of the job as an O&G registrar was delivering bad news. It was a generally positive job with very few disasters but when it went wrong it could go spectacularly wrong. It was during my time working with Nele that I would hear what I believe is the worst sound in the world – the visceral screams and cries of a woman who has lost their baby. The sound is shrill. Guttural. It cuts you to your core. We had to stay strong in front of the patient and their families because it was our job to support them in this awful time, but we were human too.

Whenever we had a foetal death in utero or a neonatal death after delivery, we were all devastated. We had usually done all we could, but it can happen so suddenly, often with a spontaneous, unavoidable cause. We always did our duty and told the family, provided support and then typically, in my experience, went into the changerooms and fell into each other's arms, debriefed and cried. *Why did this happen? It was so quick.* Sometimes there was no rhyme or reason. A complication would just occur. I always found it so difficult not to cry when we had foetal or neonatal deaths and it didn't matter how long I was in the job. I never got used to that sound of maternal grief.

When I started in general practice as a registrar, I was having so much difficulty sleeping I thought I might be depressed. Work-life balance seemed to be a distant dream, as I was working in two roles, not one. As a GP obstetric registrar, I was participating in an on-call roster and trying to learn general practice at the same time. The practice was incredibly supportive, but I was struggling with the change in roles. I had been prescribed some antidepressants, an SSRI (selective serotonin reuptake inhibitor) called citalopram, as I started to think I had a mood disorder. I was reluctant to take them and figured I would wait until I had my holidays and reassess.

I had almost finished my basic term as a GP registrar when I went on a family holiday abroad, stopping in South Korea, England, Scotland,

Ireland, France, Italy and ending in Singapore for New Year's Eve. I only got four weeks' holiday a year. To go away with the family, it needed to coincide with school holidays. We started in London, checking out all the local sites, and we were in Paris when I started thinking about this whole depression idea and discovered I just didn't feel depressed. Spending less than a week away from general practice had given me some much-needed insight into the fact that this was situational. I didn't like general practice. It felt like a machine to me, designed for income generation, not patient care. I was finding it difficult to balance my need to deliver evidence-based care, both in GP land and as a GP O&G registrar, with the need to get the billing right.

I had also spent years focused on O&G and neglecting the general body systems unless relevant to my field, so it was a steep learning curve. I remembered the guy who gave the speech on my first day at medical school and how he seemed to imply that general practice was almost the default option when you couldn't do anything else. In fact, I sensed this was a common opinion among consultants of all different fields. People with this opinion clearly never spent a day in the shoes of a general practitioner! I have nothing but admiration for anyone who can have such an effective, broad-based knowledge and skill set, deliver excellent patient care and still manage the billing. However, I knew general practice wasn't for me.

I was so happy to go back to my first love, O&G, and I felt there would be a place for me because in my absence they had frequently been short-staffed. I called the general practice I was working for from France and quit that night (daytime in Australia). I was so relieved and really enjoyed the rest of my holiday, exploring France a bit more before going to my favourite place in the world, Italy. Meandering along the narrow canals of Venice, I was in awe of this amazing place. On a gondola ride I saw the Bridge of Sighs before leaving Venice to pick up a little rental car. This was hilarious! The rental company gave us this tiny little car you could barely fit in, let alone all of us and our very Western-sized luggage.

The rental company provided an upgrade to a bigger car that just fit us and all our luggage.

On the way to Tuscany to stay in a little villa, gorgeous scenery abounded. The villa was so peaceful. While I can't remember what I needed sugar for, I do remember spending over half an hour looking for it at the local supermarket only be told it's called *zucchero*. No wonder I couldn't find it! After finally locating the sugar, I took it to the checkout only to find it was all self-service. I had never experienced anything like it! It was many years before self-service would become the norm in Australia. It was quite the novelty.

I absolutely loved planning these overseas trips, and I spent hours researching and booking them. I also made little itineraries for the kids to make it a bit more fun and so they felt included in everything. Everyone tells you not to drive in Rome but I was convinced it wouldn't be a problem, so I booked the car rental drop-off in Rome. Driving into Rome it became clear why people warned against it. The traffic was a nightmare! Unfortunately, after a few attempts it became clear the drop-off point had moved. *This wasn't in the plan.* It all seemed very funny at the time, but it lost its lustre when I realised the new drop-off was over a kilometre from the motel I had booked. My whining rivalled any dog shelter as I dragged my huge suitcase along cobblestone roads all the way to the hotel. Note to self: *Pack lighter!*

It was in Rome that I discovered and dubbed the notorious "trip step". It seemed every time we left the hotel we would see someone trip on one of the little cobblestones. This became a hilarious little challenge to see who the next victim would be of the dreaded "trip step". The holiday ended in Singapore, seeing in the new year on the roof of the Marina Bay Sands hotel, just as planned. This was the lap of luxury, and I felt like we deserved to be pampered. I have fantastic memories of this trip, and I felt like the kids were at the right age to really enjoy and remember it.

It was a great reward for a whole lot of hard work. Two of my favourite mental mantras and sayings at this time were that I needed to *fit life in between* and *I'll sleep when I'm dead.* My work schedule was full, I was fitting in whatever I could when I was off work, and I was missing so much precious time with my beautiful family, but I was so proud to be a doctor and absolutely loved my job. As a hard-working mum, I constantly felt guilty about this work ethic and did my best to find time to fit fun things in with the kids and make lasting, fond memories we could all hold on to. I often tried to fit things in no matter how tired or fatigued I was because being there for the kids was more important to me than sleep.

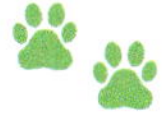

After returning from Europe, I went back to my role as an O&G registrar. I was happy to be back and decided that, since I couldn't do the training program without uprooting my family and I clearly wasn't cut out for general practice, I would just stay in this role. This was a position I could really sink my teeth into. I felt that I could update all the policies and procedures and become an asset to the department. I was also teaching the medical students, which I absolutely loved.

One of the many wonderful things about being a doctor is getting to meet some truly spectacular and wise people. One of these incredible people was a locum from India named Essa. He was a ray of sunshine and we worked hard, kept up to date and laughed together about our least favourite words in obstetrics – "dips", meaning decreases in the foetal heart rate, and "trickles", referring to maternal bleeding during or after birth. Working with Essa made every day a pleasure and he remains a dear friend. The midwives were also amazing people, many of whom became treasured friends as well as respected colleagues. We spent many days and nights together bonding over our love of family and shared experiences good and bad.

My fast-paced life forged ahead. In 2010 we went on another international holiday. I was again *fitting life in between!* I spent many months researching, planning and booking the holiday and absolutely loved this. Perhaps I was a travel agent in a previous life? I planned and booked all the segments of a wonderful holiday to Italy, Greece and Africa in December 2010. It was the trip of a lifetime. I got to go back to my favourite country, Italy, explored beautiful Greece and went on safari in Africa. I worked hard to be able to afford this trip and was only on leave for the four weeks away, so would have to go back to work as soon as I got home. This was a lot of pressure. Whenever you came off an on-call roster, it took some time for your body to adjust to normal sleep patterns, so there was a sleep debt that I just never seemed to catch up on during this holiday. I think this is probably the definition of burning the candle at both ends.

I absolutely loved seeing my children enjoy these wonderful experiences. As a normal, hard-working doctor with a family, I felt enormous guilt not being around as much because of work. Being fatigued when I was home made this guilt even worse. I tried to always let the kids know how much they meant to me, how proud I was of them, and be available for them. But by that stage, my lack of personal boundaries around rest and self-care seemed to have become the norm for all of us.

I made sure no-one thought twice about waking me up to tell me something or ask something, no matter how tired I was, and I never complained. Trying to "fit things in between" was also disrupting my rest. This, combined with my inability to set boundaries and create good sleep hygiene, made me more fatigued than most. The level of fatigue I was experiencing at this time is very difficult to explain. This goes beyond tired, beyond sleep deprived, beyond normality and beyond description. At times I found it hard to string sentences together in my time off. In my opinion, trying to fit everything in was starting to burn my body out. I just didn't recognise it at the time.

In December 2013, it was time for another overseas trip, this time to Finland. I had again really enjoyed planning this trip, but this time it was different. It didn't seem to be as enjoyable. I felt a lot of pressure to create happy family memories, had put a lot of time and effort into planning, booking and paying for this trip, but I just wasn't enjoying it and I didn't understand why. I had booked so many exciting adventures, including swimming in survival suits in the Baltic Sea, ice rally car driving, ice fishing, ice go-karting, a trip to Santa Claus Village and staying in a glass igloo. On paper, it was a dream holiday, but I just wasn't feeling it this time. I was so disappointed that I didn't seem to be able to make a good holiday happen for my family.

One night at a restaurant, around the dinner table, it all finally got the better of me. I was exhausted. I worked so hard to be able to afford it and was very much looking forward to this trip. In my eyes, this would also likely be our last international holiday together as a family so I was feeling pressure to make lasting memories. I was nostalgic and fragile. While I couldn't articulate why, I was upset, then upset with myself for ruining the night. I sobbed for a while at the dinner table, unaffected by the prying eyes of others. Upon reflection, something was already breaking in me on the inside.

Angie left for university, and after she was settled in at her new accommodation I went back to work. I couldn't believe my baby girl was leaving home. The joyous sounds of her banter and sometimes the loud sound of her playing the drums, had always filled the house, and the kids were what made this a home. Now they had both moved out and started their respective university courses, the house was very lonely and dreadfully quiet. I felt isolated and completely alone. I didn't realise it yet, but I was unravelling. All the work I had done to get here, all the sacrifices made, were about to come undone!

THE BEAST

PTSD is the beast that lives deep in my psyche,
with unfettered access to every aspect of my life

My pleas for compassion, care and rest,
an irreverent soliloquy falling on deaf ears

In silence I fade into the expansive void, my sense of self spaghettified,
like matter entering the event horizon of a black hole

What's the point in fighting it anyway? I think to myself,
as the long battle overwhelms my capacity to mount a defence

It has the upper hand, it knows my deepest fears, my darkest secrets,
and fights dirty, using them to its advantage

Still, I fight with no idea of the outcome,
buoyed by the fact that others have defeated this same beast before me

Hamstrung by my inability to use pharmaceutical means to cope,
my body and mind betray me, still I fight on

The beast lives in the depths of my soul,
no matter how many times I defeat it

It lurks around the corners of life's hardest times,
like a stealthy predator just waiting for me to fall

For now, it would seem, I have the upper hand,
my foe retreats into the shadows, waiting for its next attack

Are you ever truly free of this fiend? I contemplate,
as I plan my return to what society refers to as "reality"

Satiated by the fight itself, patiently, the beast awaits...

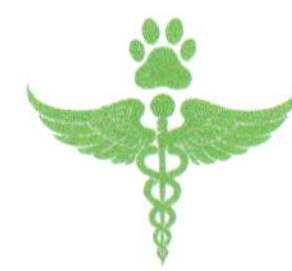

It started like any other year, but 2014 would be very different for me. Everything was changing, the kids were gone and I was more tired than ever. *Why am I struggling so much? Why are things so difficult at home?* I was finding it harder to get to sleep and every time I closed my eyes, I seemed to see disaster after disaster, waking up panicked. I didn't understand why I was feeling generally more anxious and afraid, having to check everything even more than usual and deeply worried about making a mistake.

I had read about a neonatal death following a vacuum delivery. A vacuum is a suction cup device that attaches to the baby's head to help with delivery. It had never once occurred to me that a baby might die after a vacuum delivery. Vacuum deliveries were commonplace, and I had successfully completed so many I had lost count. In this case, the baby had died as a result of resuscitation complications, not the vacuum itself, but I was so focused on not making an error that my mind immediately logged this as a risk and I suddenly became very anxious about vacuum deliveries.

I was in survival mode, and my inner critic was giving me a beating. *You need to do better, you need to take more care, the kids don't need you anymore, your husband doesn't love you, you're a terrible doctor, the world* would *be better off without you.*

My unravelling was looming and it would be very quick and very painful!

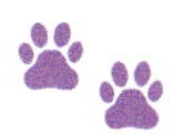

April 14, 2014, would be the day my life changed forever. This was the day I tried to make my internal pain, anxiety, fatigue and suffering stop. I really wasn't thinking logically when I took the overdose of tablets. It's hard to explain. I just thought I could make the world stop for a minute.

For the previous few months I felt like I was really struggling with exhaustion, joking with the odd colleague when we booked a theatre case that I was the one who needed the anaesthetic. It seemed every time I closed my eyes all I saw was a pool of blood, and all I felt was the overwhelming sense of personal responsibility that was now weighing me down like a concrete block chained around my neck, dragging me to the bottom of the sea. I missed the kids and the happy sounds of their laughter filling the house. I was in crisis and I was completely unaware that I wasn't coping.

I had been on call over the weekend. The next morning, as usual, I would hand over to the oncoming registrar and hope to get sleep that night. What I didn't know was that this would be the last time that my life as I knew it would ever be the same. It felt like a hard day but hard days weren't that unusual for doctors, right? There was nothing unique about it really. At the end of this day I picked up my bag, my lunch box and my bottle of water, got in the car as I usually did. It was a shiny, white Mercedes-Benz impulse buy designed to ease the pain of lost time with loved ones. I started the long drive home, sobbing all the way. I had no recollection of the drive, no idea how I got home, only recalling snippets of the journey at best. I tried to stem the tears as I drove up into the driveway of our lovely little rental home, my now adult kids both at university. I gathered myself together, forced myself to stop my blubbering and entered our little rental home.

As I walked in the door I could smell a roast chicken cooking and could see it was well underway. I had been running on autopilot since the kids left home, feeling isolated and alone. The house felt dark, cold and lonely as it had every day since my children had gone to university. I found myself feeling really negative and for some reason I had thought about hurting myself the day before. My usual practice after a weekend on call was to come home and watch some mind-numbing television. My poison of choice being Australian drama like *Neighbours* and *Home and Away*. It was the one way that I had to switch off, to stop my brain from thinking about the events of the day. But this day was different. I did go to the lounge room to sit and watch my favourite shows, but, feeling alone and miserable, I grabbed the bottle of wine from the fridge and, sobbing quietly, took myself off to the bedroom. I rifled through the bedside drawers, knowing that there were tablets somewhere but not knowing what type of pharmaceutical poison might be in there, not even putting much thought into what I might find or what it might do to me.

All I could think was: *Please let the pain stop. Please let me feel at peace. I* need *rest. MAKE IT STOP!* Nothing I had done to this point made any difference. I had tried to reduce my work hours but my financial commitments were too high. I had even changed jobs for a while but that didn't work. There was a sense of desperation in my soul. I just wanted the treadmill of life to stop! *Somebody, please make it stop* I screamed over and over in my head but to no avail. I knew what I was doing but I had no conscious control over it as I picked up the bottle of wine and poured myself another glass. I grabbed the pills from the bedside table. I now know it was citalopram. This is an antidepressant that I had in the drawer from a long time ago, when I thought I may have been depressed in general practice, but ultimately decided that it was situational and consequently had not taken them. In total I took 12 tablets of citalopram, hardly a lethal dose, but I wasn't thinking about killing myself. In fact, I don't believe I was thinking about much at all. I just wanted the pain to stop and to be able to rest. No amount of Australian TV drama was going to numb my mind enough on this day!

I lay there thinking about my life, how hard I worked to get into medicine, to pass the degree, to get to this point in my life. Having left school at 14, there didn't seem to be any expectation from family, friends or even from myself that I would be able to achieve anything academically, much less become a doctor. I had worked so hard to get where I was. *Why did I feel so bad? Why was I wanting to end it all this night?* Resilience training was a regular part of my life as a doctor and I had done my fair share. I thought I was the most resilient person I knew. *Was I wrong? Why am I the only person struggling? I'm weak, inadequate, not good enough.* Those are the words that echoed through my brain as if it were on a loudspeaker on repeat! These were familiar patterns of self-doubt that harked back to the old me but why was I feeling them again now? *They would all be better off without me!* I tried to make sense of it all as I lay there.

I started to feel very strange. I heard the dishes clanging in the distance as my husband was making dinner and I lay there thinking about how disappointed my family would be if anything happened to me. I began to think about my beautiful children, how much I loved being a mother, how much time I had lost with them because of my work ethic. How often I had missed things because I was working or so tired that I couldn't keep my eyes open. I tried wherever I could to, as I called it, "fit life in between". As a hard-working mum, I always tried to make amends for my absence with the children by being available to them no matter how fatigued I was, to help them with their homework, to watch whatever new trick they had learned, to listen to their new music or just to talk to them about their school day.

But right then, all I could think was how inadequate I was for them as a mum – *they'd be better off without me* – how I'd be leaving them behind and how they might blame themselves. I started to type a letter to them on the iPad, writing about how much I loved them, how much richness and joy they brought into my life, how much I loved being a mother and how much this would let them down. I stopped and hurriedly deleted it as dinner was coming. Tears streaming down my face, I took some time to appreciate the meal as it was placed in front of me. After about three mouthfuls though, I began to feel extremely unwell. I was nauseated, my stomach was churning, my tears were still falling, and I started to feel an overwhelming sense of dread and doom. The urgency to go to the bathroom overtook me and I jumped up, dropping the knife off the plate as I did.

The nausea and diarrhoea were incessant and unrelenting. It felt violent, almost as if it was a punishment for what I had just done, a punishment for all the wrongs I'd ever done, for all the people who might have suffered as a result of my inadequacies. The sense of doom was accompanied by a rush of blood to my head, which got worse, and I started to feel like my head was going to explode. My heart was pounding, pressure was building and I started to shake uncontrollably. It was then that I realised what I had done. I felt completely alone, like there was nobody that could help me and whatever I did next would likely only ever cause harm. However, I knew I needed help if I was going to get any better. I was so torn in my thinking between wanting all my internal pain to end and a deep sense of fear that I may actually be dying.

It's a strange sensation having done what I did, as I didn't really want to die – that wasn't the intention. The intention was purely to stop the pain, stop the roller coaster that I was on. All of a sudden, I was thinking like a medical professional. I understood that I was in trouble and I needed medical care. The time between calling the ambulance and the ambulance arriving seemed to disappear – maybe I blocked it out, perhaps it never even existed. I felt alone. It was all a blur – running to the toilet, running back, shaking, crying, the despair and the knowledge of what I had done, and how this might impact on both my career and my family, slowly sinking in.

The doctor in charge of the emergency department I attended that evening explained to me that I had a condition called serotonin syndrome where my autonomic nervous system was overactive because of serotonin toxicity caused by my overdose earlier in the evening. I had only ever read about this syndrome in medical texts so I knew it was rare. This would explain the nausea, diarrhoea, impending sense of doom and agitation. He asked if I would guarantee my safety and of course I agreed. Then he stated that if that was the case, I could be kept in overnight for observation and discharged in the morning with psychiatric follow-up. My relief at this suggestion was absolutely palpable. I was distressed and keen to avoid hospital admission. I was terrified of being reported to AHPRA (the Australian Health Practitioner Regulation Agency), aware that this was the reason many doctors in distress or with mental health issues reportedly don't disclose or seek help, and what this might mean for my career.[1] I was also absolutely exhausted. The stress on my autonomic nervous system from serotonin syndrome was starting to take a toll. Having serotonin syndrome feels like you're being chased by someone with a gun trying to kill you. It's a constant state of extreme fight or flight. I was given some sedation and finally fell asleep, with nurses frequently checking on me – the only disruption to the din of the hospital emergency department.

In the morning it was agreed I would be discharged and sent home. My heart had stopped pounding out of my chest, the diarrhoea had settled, and I was keen to get out of there. I wanted to get away from everything familiar, so I planned to leave town for a few days to see family. I went home and started packing for the trip away. I hadn't even finished packing my bag when I started to feel that same impending sense of doom, extreme flushing and pounding heart. I had been advised that if my symptoms deteriorated, I needed to come back and, while I could feel a knot in the pit of my stomach, I knew this was an indication to return. This time I was admitted for observation and cardiac monitoring until things seemed to calm down. I was discharged again the next day and finally felt that it was safe to head off as planned. Even with the drama of the last two days, I could not have predicted for a second what would happen next.

Going away to see family was the only way I could think of that may help me process what was going on. Edging closer to my destination, I was so relieved to be driving away from home and all the stress it represented, but not at all looking forward to having to talk to someone about what I had done. I was so unwell. I knew I couldn't drive myself. However, I always had trouble being a passenger in a car. This came from years of my father driving erratically as a form of control. My father had used the vehicle as a weapon several times in my childhood, threatening to drive into a pole or give me something to be frightened of by driving erratically. Several times when he fought with my mother in the car, he threatened to run us off the road and even swerved at times, laughing to himself as if it was a big joke while I squealed in terror.

This was an anxiety I just couldn't control, so it didn't matter who was at the wheel. I guess it could be perceived as if I were criticising people's driving skills when this anxiety would consume me, but I knew full well that this was *my* problem and had always taken responsibility for it. However, this day was different, and my autonomic nervous system was on fire. It didn't matter how hard I tried – I couldn't reign in the severe anxiety I felt as a passenger when the car overtook that large truck on the highway. This wasn't just anxiety; this was serotonin syndrome. I needed medical attention, and I needed it now! That blue and white hospital sign was a beacon of hope. This is where you met me in the first pages of this book.

Once I'd been admitted to the emergency department and was aware of the gravity of the situation, my family were contacted and made their way in to see me. I decided in my wisdom that, for now, I would just tell the children I'd had a reaction to medication. Having a medical background, I understood that having a family member who had attempted or completed suicide would increase a child's own risk of suicide. I so desperately wanted to do the right thing and protect my children from this potential risk. In hindsight, I can see that this was a mistake because I lied, but at the time I truly felt that I was doing the right thing by them.

The doctor who admitted me seemed, at the time, sympathetic to my plight, referring to me as a "junior doctor in distress". Dr Hartwell was a very tall, middle-aged woman who had an air of confidence about her. The years of experience in medicine were etched in the little wrinkles that gently framed her face. She was gentle, caring and supportive of my needs. She was concerned about my mental welfare and made me assure my safety overnight. While I agreed to remain safe, it was something I was finding desperately difficult. I was now convinced my career was over, my children would no longer respect me when they found out what I had done, my family would be disappointed in me, and any road back would be almost impossible. *They're all better off without me!* I became acutely suicidal as the evening hours passed. In the morning, I admitted to that senior doctor I had contemplated using the bottle of potassium that was in my bedside drawer overnight to kill myself.

The admission of this fact seemed to ruin our therapeutic relationship. Dr Hartwell seemed visibly concerned, expressing it was against protocol to have someone acutely suicidal admitted to the ward. It appeared to me that her polite, caring, supportive demeanour completely changed. She now seemed desperate to offload me to a mental health facility, her preferred one being a local, private mental health care unit. What I failed to appreciate at the time is that the toll of the past few months, of being on autopilot and my illness, seemed to be having an impact on other relationships as well. She referred me to her preferred psychiatrist who would accept my admission.

As a clinician, I had heard from several patients about how disempowering it is to be on the other side of medicine. I had experienced being a patient before with the birth of both my children, several childhood illnesses, and an admission for anaphylaxis in my early 20s. I was about to learn firsthand what it felt like to be completely disempowered. I was a long way from home, feeling vulnerable and very unwell, so I was relieved to be admitted and get the help that I knew I desperately needed. The serotonin syndrome had finally settled, and I was prepared for what work I needed to do to get better. I was referred to a psychiatrist for treatment. From the outset, this consultation left me feeling dismissed and unheard at a time when I was acutely unwell and vulnerable. She diagnosed me with depression, suggested I start on an antidepressant closely related to the one that had caused the serotonin syndrome in the first place.

The diagnosis came as no surprise and I accepted this as gospel. However, based on my medical training and my recent experience, the choice of medication frightened me. I raised my concerns, explaining that the similarity between the drugs felt unsafe to me, but I did not feel those concerns were meaningfully addressed or explored. I may have been unwell at the time but I was still an intelligent, up-to-date doctor. I understood the risks as I saw them but didn't feel confident in my ability to advocate for myself, nor did I feel supported in doing so. When I hesitated, I felt significant internal pressure to proceed and was reassured that starting on a reduced dose would be safe, even if the symptoms returned. I reluctantly agreed, reasoning that she would be in a better position to make this decision for me rather than myself right now. This would be one of my greatest lessons in life – how vital it is for me to listen to my instincts.

Within about 36 hours of starting this medication, I was symptomatic again with serotonin syndrome. When I talked to the pharmacy where they dispensed the medications, they informed me there was a discrepancy between the dose I believed I had agreed upon and what I had been given. My blood pressure and heart rate again began to rise, and I developed my old friend, diarrhoea. I asked to see the doctor and this time stood firm in refusing to continue the medication. I discussed with her what the plan would be now. Her plan was to discharge me with no medication to allow it to 'wash out' of my system. The expectation being that I would organise my own follow-up closer to home. I was profoundly unwell, frightened and increasingly destabilised.

It would be less than a week before I was acutely suicidal again and voluntarily readmitted to another private inpatient mental health care facility, this time of my choosing, closer to home called Healing House. Looking back, the sequence of events felt dangerous. I had been discharged into the community without adequate support at a time of significant risk. This experience was not about one clinician or one decision. It was a stark reflection of a mental health system under enormous strain. Mental health systems are overloaded; there aren't enough beds for patients and the stigma around mental health can be a barrier to people (particularly doctors) accessing appropriate support, contributing to poor treatment outcomes. I feel like I was left out in the world, flailing, desperately unwell and without the help I needed. The outcome could have been very different had I not known what to do. I sought my own support because I knew how to, where to, and I could afford it. So many others aren't so lucky.

The admission to Healing House would be the turning point in my mental health struggles. When I was first admitted, as is standard practice, I wasn't allowed to have contact with the external world and I wasn't allowed to leave. That was just fine with me. I didn't want to go anywhere, I didn't want to see anyone and I definitely didn't want to do anything. In this facility, I felt that I was being cared for by somebody who cared about the outcome for me. I was having severe problems with sleep, with recurrent nightmares, which I would come to understand much later to be a symptom of PTSD (Post Traumatic Stress Disorder). They gave me something to help me sleep, and I started regular cognitive behavioural therapy and regular consultations with the psychiatrist. I was reluctant to leave my room even after the restrictions had been lifted, as I didn't want to run into anyone I knew now I was closer to home.

There were several very significant turning points in my life that occurred during my time at Healing House, the first of which being some fantastic advice from my amazing mother. On one of her many visits, my mother sat down and discussed some of the hardships that she had faced in her life. Mum had always been a tower of strength to me. She had survived all manner of abuse, had the strength to run her own businesses, and faced any hardship head on. I always thought I was the most resilient person I knew but there's only so far that resilience can take you. Mum agreed and she talked to me about how she'd suffered some significant work-related issues that pretty much ended her career but she never did anything about it and this was one of her biggest regrets. She talked about how this impacted on her life and that she wished she had sought the help she needed. Her compassion, care and understanding were just what I needed at that time. I took this great piece of advice and embraced the treatment plan with both arms. I wanted to get better and return to function.

The second fantastic piece of advice I received came from the exercise physiologist who optimistically arrived on the ward every morning with a pep in his step and an encouraging, uplifting, almost musical voice to get us up and moving. Despite some recent weight loss, at 164 centimetres, I was still classified as morbidly obese at the time, weighing in at 108 kilograms, and the last thing I wanted to do was leave the facility for fear of being seen by someone I knew. However, one day after I refused to get up and asked him how on Earth it would help me, he made a statement that would change the course of my life.

He said, and I quote, "It's simple. It's a choice. You can choose to sit here or you can choose to get up and live."

To begin with, I was quite affronted by this statement. *How dare he think that this was a choice!* I contemplated his statement deeply, delving into the depths of my soul to check its validity. This is something I had been doing a lot with the cognitive behavioural therapy, checking validity. He was right. Whether or not I got up and participated was a choice. After much thought, I also came to the deep realisation that my current reality came about because of a series of choices that I made. I couldn't blame anyone for the situation I was in because I chose it! I began to see then that I could make different choices and create a different reality. The very next time his joyous voice came to get us all up to move, I rose from my chair, and I chose life!

Sadly, the last significant turning point at Healing House wasn't a positive one. Early in my admission I was started on a low dose of one of the most commonly used and well-tolerated SSRI's, fluoxetine. I had been presented with a series of options but many of them had weight gain as a potential side effect, something I really wanted to avoid since I'd started becoming physically active and losing weight. In the end, I chose to trial a very low dose of fluoxetine as I was unlikely to gain weight on this drug. I was stabilised on this very low dose of fluoxetine but as the dose was increased, sadly, I developed side effects again.

Very quickly after increasing the dose, I again developed serotonin syndrome symptoms but this time it also damaged my liver. My anxiety was at an all-time high, my heart was racing, my blood pressure was elevated and my old friend, diarrhoea, was back for another visit! I developed medical anorexia, not the disorder but the medical term 'anorexia', referring to the loss of appetite, which was ironic given how overweight I was. I was in hospital for so long I'd forgotten what day it was. I was unable to eat even the simplest of foods without upsetting my stomach significantly and developing severe intractable diarrhoea. I overheard discussions suggesting these symptoms might be psychosomatic (caused by the mind), something I found confronting considering how physically unwell I was. There seemed to be some surprise when a scan revealed that I had a nonspecific inflammation of my stomach lining and colon (gastritis and colitis) as well as some signs of acute liver damage.

My health rapidly deteriorated. After 14 days of no nutrition and a bout of metabolic acidosis, I was a mess. It felt like "It's all in your head", had become a familiar refrain, once I had a documented mental health history. I was weak, sick, malnourished, exhausted and felt completely alone. I was struggling to eat anything and in the end a tube was placed down my nose and into my stomach. This is now on the list of things I never want to experience again. The tube felt enormous and as it passed down the back of my throat it got stuck several times. I had to sip water to push it past any resistance and with my ongoing nausea this made me feel like vomiting. After the tube was inserted, I successfully advocated for my own transfer to a bigger hospital for further investigation and treatment since, despite excellent care at this hospital, I didn't seem to be getting any better. I was transferred to a much larger facility near my children, and they were there to greet me when I arrived.

It was so lovely to see their smiling faces, and I no longer felt alone. In this hospital I would undergo a liver biopsy that would confirm that I had a drug-induced liver injury, likely secondary to the fluoxetine. They stopped trying to feed me and rested my gut for 48 hours. It would take months to recover from this liver injury and the impact that it had on my gastrointestinal system. I was told that my options for an antidepressant were extremely limited given the reactions that I had, and it would be wise to consider natural ways to manage my depression and anxiety. I finally began to see a light at the end of the tunnel. I felt like I might be able to start to recover now – but I was definitely wrong!

After a few days I was able to eat a few morsels of food. I drank ginger beer to up the calorie intake to ensure that I didn't get hypoglycaemia (low blood sugar). This was a big hospital so beds came at a premium and they seemed keen to discharge me once I was feeling better and could eat. I had been given some pain relief and anti-nausea medications after the biopsy and was finally discharged. I was keen to get home and start the process of getting well. I was so grateful for the care I received at this hospital. My hopes were dashed when about an hour's drive from home my symptoms returned. Once again, I was extremely unwell with serotonin syndrome but this time it was unclear how I could possibly have it since I had stopped the drug that caused it.

When you have serotonin syndrome you're agitated, anxious, hypervigilant and extremely unwell. When it became clear how unwell I was again, we stopped at the next town. I was admitted to yet another hospital, this time a little hospital an hour from my home. My blood pressure was again dangerously high, my heart was pounding out of my chest and I had a low-grade temperature. My old friend, diarrhoea, came back with a vengeance, and I started to wonder if I was going to ever recover. I asked if I could be transferred back to Dr Hartwell, the doctor I had met in an earlier admission, as I felt that she may still have some compassion for my situation and seemed to know what to do to support serotonin syndrome. The lovely people at this little hospital took great care of me and, upon my request, organised my transfer. Dr Hartwell accepted me back for which I was very grateful. Only later would I reflect on how my earlier psychiatric experience may have influenced how vulnerable and guarded I felt during this admission.

My admission was lengthy and difficult. As a medical professional myself, I'm quite sure I was a difficult patient and my clinical progress had been slow. When my liver function tests finally turned in the right direction, I was discharged. Before I left, I discussed with the pharmacist my concerns over developing serotonin syndrome symptoms despite stopping the SSRI that caused them. We both had a look at the literature and discovered that fluoxetine was notorious for taking a long time to wash out of the body and can (rarely) cross-react with the medications I was given after the liver biopsy. I developed the opinion that what I had been experiencing was a garden variety case of, you guessed it, serotonin syndrome. I felt a degree of vindication, finally understanding that what I had been experiencing had a rare but physiological explanation. However, at the same time I understood that serotonin syndrome had made me look and behave somewhat neurotic. As doctors I think we all understand that we make terrible patients. I think I was perhaps the worst! I was constantly reading to try to understand what was going on in my body and to make sense of a situation that seemed to be endless. By the time I was discharged it felt like both Dr Hartwell and I shared the relief that my condition was finally improving.

My son, Eliot, was going on an overseas trip and I was able to be discharged just in time to see him off at the airport and then go home. I'd been sick for so long I didn't know what home was and I certainly wasn't looking forward to fighting my way back to health. There were a lot of formalities required in order to return to work. I steadily chipped away at each and every one with fierce dedication to the task at hand, ever mindful of protecting my mental health. I would have to be cleared by an AHPRA-accredited forensic psychiatrist before I could return to work. It was suggested that I might have an adjustment disorder that caused the depression. Anyone who has ever had to return to work after illness or injury would know there's a process and it takes time. It would take another three months, a hell of a lot of fighting my symptoms and illness, and a demanding series of clearances to finally get back to work. In December 2014, with my head held high, I returned to work not knowing what would lie ahead. I felt like I had achieved the impossible and I felt no shame for what had occurred. *I survived*. I was back to functionality, loud and proud!

THE DARKNESS INSIDE

Darkness falls, indiscriminately taking all it can along the way
There's nowhere left to run, hope fades, there's nothing left to say
Sorrow's shadow descends like a tempest, you can't outrun it, don't even try
The darkness doesn't care about the people it hurts or how much you cry
No-one is exempt from its grasp, regardless of sex, race or age
Getting angry or sad doesn't help, it just fuels its relentless rage
Some seem to overcome it with the help of those they love
But for others the darkness takes them to the
brink, giving them an impolite shove
For those taken by the darkness, the suffering may now be over
But for those left behind they may never feel true closure
There's a place deep inside only the darkness seems to reach
It sets up a defence there even those close to you find hard to breach
I've come to learn that fighting the darkness is really done alone
Only from the inside can its power be truly overthrown
So, I say to the darkness, "Go away and leave me in peace,
I may not have much left to lose but please let the suffering cease"
The darkness has come for me again, but this time I will stand strong
Knowing I had what I needed to fight it within me all along

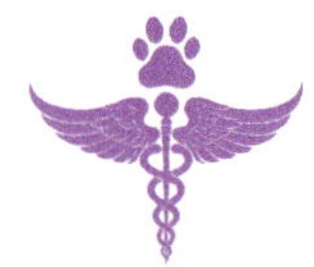

It took several months to settle back into working full-time. I had spent eight months in intensive therapy, learning how my thoughts, feelings and behaviours were linked, learning what my core beliefs were, how my choices and lack of healthy boundaries contributed to my mental health struggles, and how important these boundaries were to healthy relationships.

At the end of the year I had the great pleasure of attending Eliot's university graduation. As I sat there in the crowd of proud parents, I was taken back to his early childhood when I made a promise that he would grow up safe, secure and knowing he was loved. I never pressured my kids to study but I guess they grew up in a household that normalised academic performance. Even still, I always told the kids I would be happy with whatever they chose to do in their lives as long as it made them happy. After feeling a wave of pride in his amazing achievements, it occurred to me that I had achieved my ultimate goal. My children were both really in the adult world now. They had grown up safe, knew that they were loved, and their lives felt secure. There was a moment of pride that, while unsaid, was palpable. Then tears overcame me. As they streamed uncontrollably down my face, I thought: *What if I had died in April? I would have missed this amazing opportunity. What would his graduation have been like for him if his mum died? I could have ruined it all for my family. How irresponsible that would have been! How much harder must his last year of university been because of my illness.* I didn't know it at the time but I was beginning to feel a deep sense of maternal guilt that would stay with me for a long time to come.

It was with a newfound knowledge of my own inner workings and a new skill set that I approached the next stage of my life. Unfortunately, when you change how you behave and how you interact with others, I believe it often creates difficulty in relationships. During this time, I was using health and fitness to cope with any stress I might experience. My new family holiday focus would be a physical challenge. I was researching, planning and training for a beautiful, six-day (and night), 70-kilometre walk called the Overland Track in Tasmania. I was controlling my food, had converted to a vegan diet and was exercising every opportunity I could. I was using mindfulness (being consciously aware of the sensations in the moment) while exercising and this was really helping me to balance the stresses at work and home. Once again, I revelled in choosing, planning, booking and preparing for this trip.

In January, our family left for the Overland Track walk in Tasmania. It was gruelling! In the first couple of days I developed blisters on my toes, which were incredibly painful. About halfway through the walk I met a lady who helped me tie the laces to avoid blisters and strap my sore toes. I hadn't realised that the blow-up pillows were made of latex (I'm allergic) and my face had swollen up with my eyes barely visible, so I didn't have a pillow either, something else to complain about. I looked like I lost a fight with Mike Tyson and my toes looked like they'd turned into a painful version of bubble wrap! It had become so unpleasant that at the halfway point we half-jokingly contemplated being airlifted out or turning back. It was exhausting and I was starving as the food provided was barely enough to survive off. I looked at the map and let everyone know it would be quicker to walk out than go back. From that point onwards, Angelina became our anchor! She knew the way out, kept us motivated and moving forward, stopped everyone from whingeing and got us to the end.

I breathed a sigh of relief and vowed to never go hiking like that again! I was so inspired by Angelina on this trip, with her resilience, leadership and tenacity making this an amazing experience for us all. I made so many rookie hiking errors. The backpacks were 18 to 20 kilograms, with way too many extras, the shoes I wore weren't properly run in, and for my first hiking experience this was a difficult starting point. Although this was a really challenging walk, I still have very fond memories of this time off grid, in nature with my beautiful children. I loved organising and making these holidays happen. I didn't know it then, but this would be the last time I would holiday with my little family.

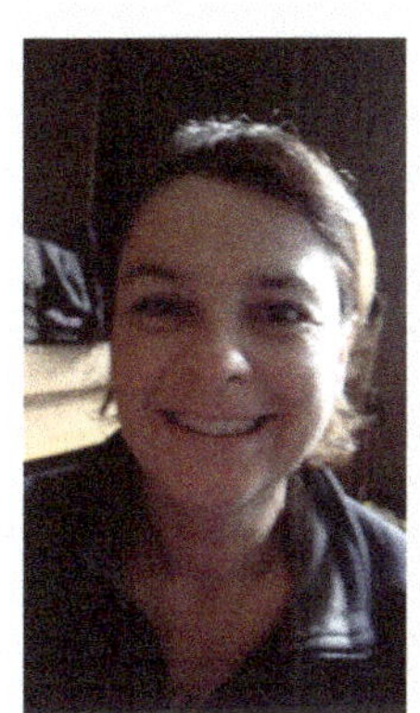

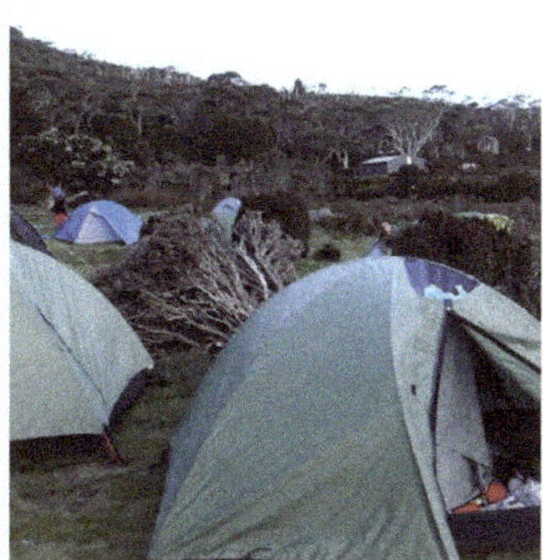

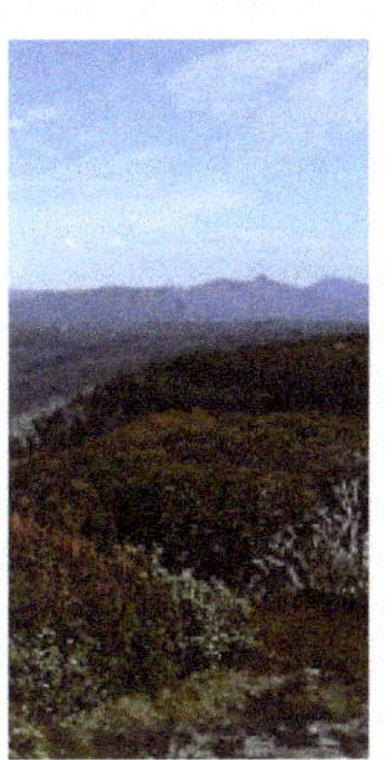

The overland track

After the walk I was still very keen to keep up my fitness. I was now a very healthy weight and keen to stay that way. I had developed an interest in triathlons and, at the age of 43, I learnt how to swim. I started riding a bike, swimming and running, and entered several small events. While I wasn't good at any of the elements, I really enjoyed these events and worked up to the Forster Ultimate triathlon, a half Ironman distance triathlon. This would involve a 1.9-kilometre swim, a 90-kilometre bike ride and a half marathon. After completing my first half marathon, I decided to keep training and register for the Forster Ultimate event. At this event, I was very slow. Thankfully, they kept the finish line open for me and at eight hours and 45 minutes I crossed the line. I had completed this gruelling endurance event. I always dreamed of being fit and healthy but struggled with my weight since childhood. This was a sweet victory. I felt the rush and, ready for more, I started to train for the full Ironman event, which included a four-kilometre swim, 180-kilometre bike ride and full marathon, to be held in Port Macquarie in 2017. Eliot agreed to join me and we started training for the Ironman event.

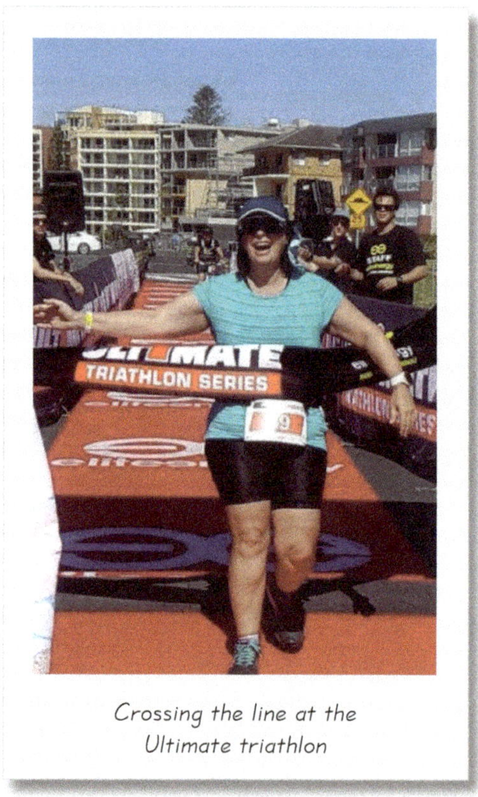

Crossing the line at the Ultimate triathlon

I was vulnerable and needed good sleep to recover while attempting to reintegrate into the working environment. The workplace was very supportive around my return to work. However, I needed a change and eventually decided to apply for another job, in another hospital, in another town so I could have a fresh start in a new environment. This time the job would be an administrative role supporting other junior doctors. I managed to secure a part-time role in teaching and support for trainees (doctors in a training program), an area that I now felt very passionately about. This would allow me to finally reduce my workload to part-time.

Before relocating for this job, Angie graduated from university. What an amazing achievement; I was so proud! Angie had always worked hard and seemed to really enjoy what she was doing. Again, sitting in the hall as a proud mum, I thought about the impact it must have had on her when I was unwell and how different things could have been had I died in 2014. Things had changed so much for my little family and there were more changes on the horizon.

I set about moving for this new job. For financial reasons, it was essential for me to take on another part-time role as an O&G registrar. This was a busy hospital. I was very nervous about this role and how I could maintain balance now with two jobs. I didn't feel like I had any choice as I had bills to pay.

I started and absolutely loved my primary role, which involved providing functional, professional and personal support as well as education for the trainees. This workplace was very supportive and had a lovely culture. The education I was providing involved a lot of simulated training scenarios and I loved teaching, so this was very fulfilling. I felt like I found my new calling. I had to start in the O&G part of the role and fairly quickly I could feel that pressure and terrible anxiety returning.

However, I reasoned this was such a supportive environment, I was well so I'd be okay. I started to have difficulty sleeping again, being recurrently woken by nightmares. Sometimes they were just your garden variety nightmare about being attacked or chased but some were more distressing, involving routine things but with bad outcomes, like emergency Caesarean sections, bleeding that wouldn't stop, resuscitations that didn't go so well. I very quickly realised I needed to get out of this additional O&G role.

Around the same time, I also started to feel like my relationship was coming to an end. I had seen firsthand the impact being a doctor could have on relationships, never thinking for a second it would happen to me. From my perspective, the realisation my decades-long relationship was over was incredibly painful and left me utterly devastated, but I knew there was no coming back.

In hindsight, the stress of moving, starting a new job, and starting a second job would have all been taking their toll on my relationships. I would eventually recognise that my mental health was again deteriorating and what I was really dealing with was PTSD. Once I was on my own, I came to understand just how precarious my personal financial position was. It was far worse than I had realised. All of the financial commitments I was personally responsible for – rent, bills, the car loan and multiple credit cards – amounted to approximately $5,500 per month. The pressure to maintain a high income suddenly felt relentless. While I was unwell, I hadn't been caring much about finances. I just took no notice. Survival took priority. In addition, I feel like when you're really stressed, the way I was when I was very sick, you spend more money on things you wouldn't usually buy. Financial strain became yet another layer of pressure on my already fragile recovery.

While all this was going on, I was still training for Ironman. I was using exercise to cope with my stress, and the need for physical activity was ever increasing as the stress and pressure built. Eliot was also training with me at the time. On one of our many very long training rides, we hit the proverbial wall! We were doing a six-hour ride to prepare and we had been going back and forth past one another for hours, eating our boiled, salted potatoes, and drinking our electrolytes. We were constantly niggling at each other not to cut corners or to pedal a certain way, and at one point we stopped and both just cried for no reason. We looked at each other, shared a hug, and mused over how tough this was and how exhausted we both were. This kind of training takes you to your limits and then sometimes pushes you past them; that's one of the reasons it can be so therapeutic. This was one of those times.

We had a chat about stopping and mutually agreed we had to continue, so we got back on our trusty triathlon bikes and finished the training ride. We reasoned that we would experience worse on the day and had to be able to push past it. Training with Eliot for Ironman was one of the most wonderful memories I have of our relationship. We really bonded over these difficult times and gave each other the strength to push past them.

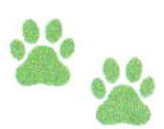

Two weeks before Ironman, I had just completed an iron infusion and was stationary at the lights when I was hit from behind at speed by another car. The impact pushed me into the car in front of me, which also pushed it into the next car. I got out of the car and after assessing the situation I realised the driver appeared to be having a seizure at the wheel. I immediately switched modes and rendered assistance. A bystander (also a nurse – what are the odds?) and I turned off her car and kept her safe until the ambulance came. I was finally able to stop and take in what had just happened. I was sore and the beautiful Mercedes I was driving was looking pretty ordinary.

I had a love-hate relationship with this car. I loved the first Mercedes I bought and had almost paid it off, but I didn't love this one as the upgrade represented a huge debt, adding to my financial pressures. Having said that, I was very grateful to be in this car for this accident as it had a head airbag, which had deployed. Even so, my neck was very sore. After looking at the carnage, the tow truck driver gave me some sage advice: "You might feel okay now but if you're sore in the morning go to the doctor and get it looked at and get the injury documented."

The next morning, just as the lovely tow truck driver had suggested, I was in a lot of pain, both in my neck and upper back. I had torn some

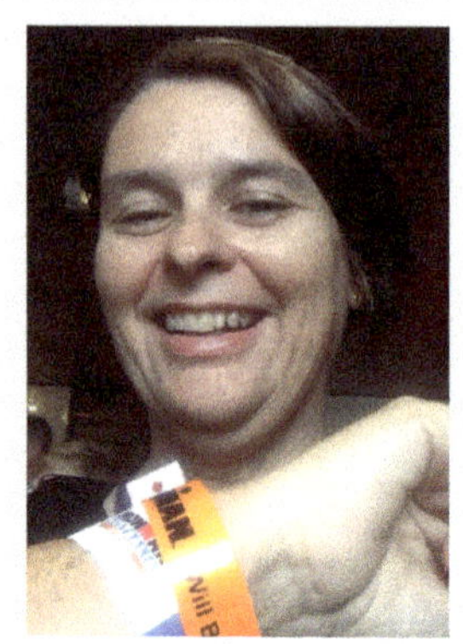
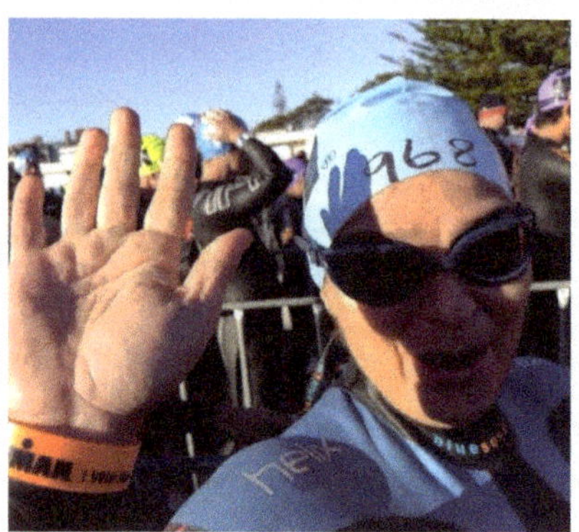

Making it to the Ironman start line

ligaments and would need physiotherapy. I looked into the cost and sought some legal advice as the treatment would be expensive. I worked on getting the third-party insurer to cover this cost for me. I had extensive physio and converted my training into low resistance, mostly in the pool, for the last two weeks of Ironman training. When I arrived at Ironman, I realised I had expended all my energy getting to the start line.

I didn't have the best start as my bike had a flat tyre that had to be fixed before the race even started. The swim was very difficult for me as my neck was so sore from the crash. I was second last out of the swim and very slow on the bike; my neck was throbbing. I remained unwavering. *You have to keep going. You've got this.*

Penny, my beautiful triathlon bike (it cost me a pretty penny)

Despite having had the bike serviced not once but twice, I continued to experience mechanical problems during the race. The chain on the bike kept coming off and I repeatedly had to stop to fix it, so I was slower than usual. Around 110 kilometres into the bike leg, I was taken off for being too slow. I was devastated. When the man put the bike on his ute, he noticed that the whole front fork was very loose and told me how lucky I was not to come off. I was doing 62 kilometres per hour down those massive hills, so it didn't bear thinking about what could have happened! I was sore, sorry for myself and defeated. *This doesn't even feel like a good training day. I have so much more in the tank. Stupid bike!* I was also thinking how things happen for a reason and perhaps being taken off saved me from an awful crash. I used the fuel I still had to cheer on Eliot and he finished just before the cutoff time. We had spent countless hours training together and while I was disappointed for myself earlier, I was very proud of his achievement!

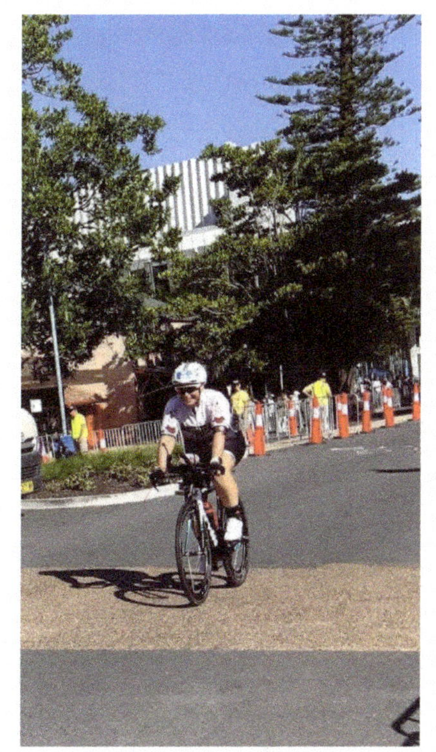

Mum took this photo while cheering me on in the bike leg

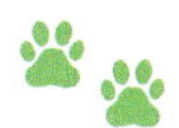

I needed to continue to maintain my ridiculous financial commitments. To do this, I had to keep the O&G job even though I was concerned that having a second job might all be too much for me to cope with. I was also under a lot of pressure and didn't know how to get myself out of the financial mess I was in.

One night, in the middle of a very busy birthing unit in this incredibly supportive environment, there were two patients about to deliver who were likely to require an assisted delivery (usually a vacuum). This was a frequent occurrence, so nothing unusual for a busy unit. I went to the first room and much to my relief I only needed to make a small cut (episiotomy) in order to facilitate the delivery. However, when I raced to the second room it was a completely different scenario. This would require an instrumental delivery, and all my anxieties, fears, worries and concerns converged in one moment. I froze just as I entered the room. Thankfully, the consultant was also present and stepped in immediately. I was frozen. Numb. I couldn't move. It was as if I was suddenly outside my body, looking down at the room from above. I could hear the sound of the baby's heart beating from the monitor, see the midwife trying to engage me and, quickly realising that I was no help, moving on to the consultant. I still couldn't move. I couldn't speak but I was aware of what was going on around me. The consultant completed the delivery that was required with ease, even taking time to teach a medical student in the process. There was no emergency, no threat, but my body had told me otherwise. I felt humiliated, useless and defeated.

I'm not sure how long it took me to come out of this dissociative state, but it was long enough for the baby to be crying and safely delivered into its mother's arms. There were no complications and there had been no delay in the delivery because the consultant was there. However, I came to the devastating realisation that I could no longer work in medicine. This was the first time I had ever experienced a dissociative episode, and I knew that this made me an unacceptable risk to my patients. My lifetime load of trauma had hit the invisible threshold beyond which I could no longer function.

I went to the bathroom and cried, then gathered myself together, spoke to the consultant and asked to be removed from the rest of the shift as I wasn't feeling well. Then I walked to the office and asked the head of department to remove me from the roster entirely. I was heartbroken. I was so passionate about my job and had always felt privileged to be a doctor. Just as I had known with my relationship, I knew that there was no coming back from this. At the end of that shift, I sat in my car in the car park of the hospital and cried uncontrollably. It was loud and ugly, and I felt the grief of the situation so viscerally. *It's over!* My inability to cope (what I now know to be PTSD) had ended my career and I wasn't sure what else I could do with myself. I was trained for one thing. I had no other significant qualifications or skills. This was my whole life!

I had spent 20 years of my life either working towards this or working within this system. I didn't know how to do anything else. I was angry at the world. Angry at myself for not being able to just cope with the stress. I was also again contemplating ending my life. *What's the point? I can't even work anymore, I'm useless to my profession, and my kids would be better off without me anyway. I've become a burden to everyone. My marriage is over, I'm on the brink financially and now I'm going to lose everything.*

I knew this inner demon well and I had beaten it before. What people don't tell you is that once your brain has seriously contemplated suicide as an option or your body has attempted to use it as a solution, it can become the default mode for critical negative situations in life. I couldn't believe I was back there! As part of my recovery in 2014, I had written an emergency plan for a situation just like this. I decided it was time to enact this emergency plan.

I called the inpatient psychiatric facility I had previously been admitted to (Healing House) and asked to be admitted again under my private health insurance. I had been working on a new model of orientation for the next cohort of trainees, and I arranged my admission for the next

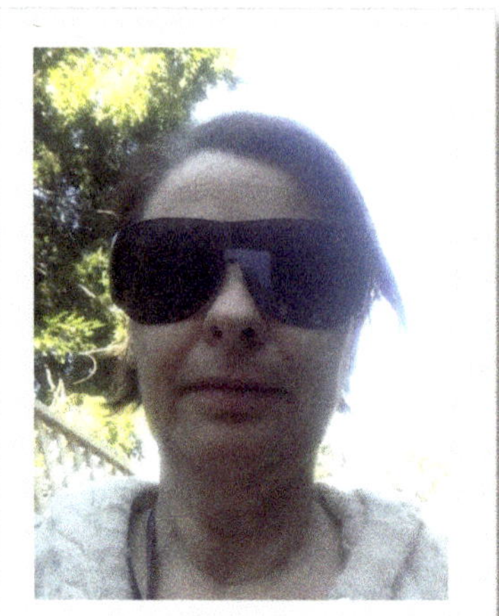
Selfie for Mum - at Healing House

day. I attended this orientation knowing I would be resigning and being admitted to an inpatient facility the next day. I gave everything I had to make this new cohort of doctors' orientation an enjoyable experience and made sure I emphasised self-care as my parting gift to a profession I loved. I enacted my safety plan, removed all means of self-harm from the house, and got myself ready to be admitted.

After I was admitted to Healing House, I was formally assessed and the psychiatrist told me, "I think you have PTSD."

I had assumed this was just a recurrence of depression, but as they were talking I realised I had *all* the symptoms of PTSD. It was one of those "aha" moments – the last few years of my life suddenly made sense! *That's why I kept having nightmares, why I can't sleep, why I relapse as soon as I'm exposed to a stressor. This explains the flashbacks to traumatic events in my life, the constant worry and irritability, the overwhelming sense of threat where there was none. It is an old foe. I get it now.*

I now live in peace with my PTSD but I was lucky to survive my suicide attempt, given that female doctors reportedly have a markedly higher rate of suicide compared with the general population.[2] This is a sobering reality for women in the health profession.

It was during this admission that I became familiar with what I affectionately refer to now as "lost days". These were days when my mood was so low I simply couldn't function. Getting out of bed to go to the toilet was difficult, so there was no chance of getting anything done on these days. Sometimes I would have several lost days in a row and then all of a sudden, without notice, I would wake up one day and feel different. I couldn't tell you what changed or why I felt different. One day could be dark and lost, and the next day could feel okay. I have come to understand that this is a way for my nervous system to reset. My brain needed these lost days to rest and recuperate so that I could hope for something different. I now refer to it as needing "autonomic downtime" and whenever my body tells me I need it I now listen.

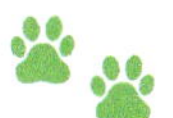

My finances were still appalling. In total, I learnt that my personal debt was over $187,000 with a car loan and lots of credit cards, but absolutely nothing to show for it. I had discussed this with Mum over the phone and we talked about my options. I could claim hardship, refinance, sell the car, or go into a debt agreement. If none of that worked, I would potentially have to go bankrupt. There are several firms out there that can assist with financial hardships like this, so I contacted one for some advice and set about trying to sort out my financial situation as, without a job, I would no longer be able to satisfy my creditors every month.

I sought financial advice and tried to figure out what to do with payment plans and financial hardship agreements. If I couldn't get on top of it all, I would have to go bankrupt, which I knew had dreadful consequences. I soldiered on and continued to struggle with the ongoing pressure from finance companies and creditors, organising meetings with them and staving them off from my hospital bed.

Mum came to visit me while I was admitted. She sat down with me and gave me the second-best piece of advice I ever got.

"It's going to be really hard to do something new in your life but I know you can. Perhaps you need to consider what else you might like to do."

She went on gently, "I've been looking into getting an assistance dog for myself and I think it might help you too. An assistance dog can help support you emotionally and help you while you get back on your feet."

She went on to explain all the research she had done about assistance dogs and how they can help people with PTSD. She'd also brought a pen and pad with her, and we sat and brainstormed what other things I may be able to do with my life.

I was sobbing, "But I worked *so* hard to get here, Mum, and I know what it takes to come back from this. I'm not sure I have it left in me!" In that moment she was just like Lois had been years earlier in the STEPS course, resolute in her belief in me.

She said, "Jodi, you *will* survive this and you *will* go on to do something else. I know you can do it! Look what you have achieved in your life." Before she left, with my permission, Mum also took the time to talk to my psychologist and get some advice on how she could best support me. This really brought home to me how much she cared.

After she left, I considered carefully what she had said. I decided not to focus on what I would do with my life at this point, since all that did was make me focus on what I had lost. Instead, I would focus on this assistance dog thing. I spent the last couple of weeks of my hospital stay planning what breed I would get, learning how I would train the dog, looking into what was required to get or accredit an assistance dog, and making a plan.

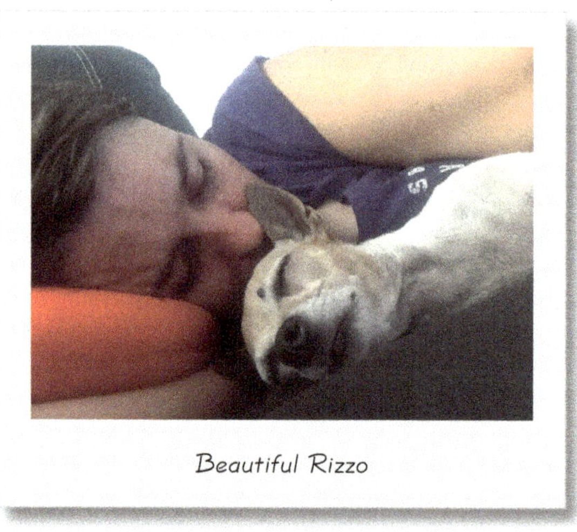

Beautiful Rizzo

All the information I was reading said you shouldn't have other dogs while training an assistance dog but I still had a family dog, Rizzo, who was now nine years old. Mum was right. Even the thought of having an assistance dog to train was making me feel better. I had the possibility of a future and even that was more than I hoped for at the time. Getting and training an assistance dog would become my new focus in life and it would, in fact, save my life!

STIGMA

S is for sad, what you said I can't forget
T is for tears that have made my face wet
I is for ignorance, if you only knew what it took
G is for grotesque, how this behaviour makes you look
M is for mean, the way you treat me is a big deal
A is for angry because stigma won't help me heal

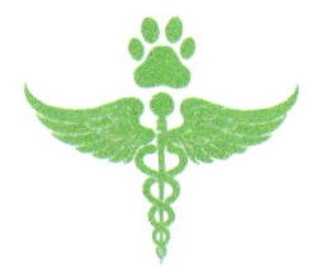

There's a lot to consider when choosing an assistance dog prospect. Is the breed easy to train? Will their energy levels fit my lifestyle? Is the breed associated with any potential serious illnesses? Can I take care of the dog and its needs? After much deliberation, I decided on a German Shorthaired Pointer (GSP) for my assistance dog. I was very active physically, this was a very intelligent breed and my daughter had two of these dogs that were beautiful animals. As if by fate, the litter of GSPs I applied for was born on the same day I had called to arrange my admission in 2017. I saw the pictures and fell in love with one of the female puppies because she had a letter 'L' in white on her forehead, but the breeder was adamant another male puppy would be a better fit because of its temperament. I named my new dog Ben after the song by Michael Jackson, as the lyrics held great meaning for me.

Ben, the two of us need look no more
We both found what we were looking for
With a friend to call my own
I'll never be alone

I just needed to wait for him to be old enough to come home. I was still trying to figure out what to do with Rizzo as the kids seemed understandably upset at the idea of her finding a new home. At the last minute the breeder decided the female with the 'L' on her forehead would be a better fit after all. As a result, the beautiful Ben became Benedicta (Benni for short). On October 6, 2017, Benni came to live with me and Rizzo. I distinctly remember picking her up from the airport. I anxiously waited for them to bring her out to me, my heart bursting

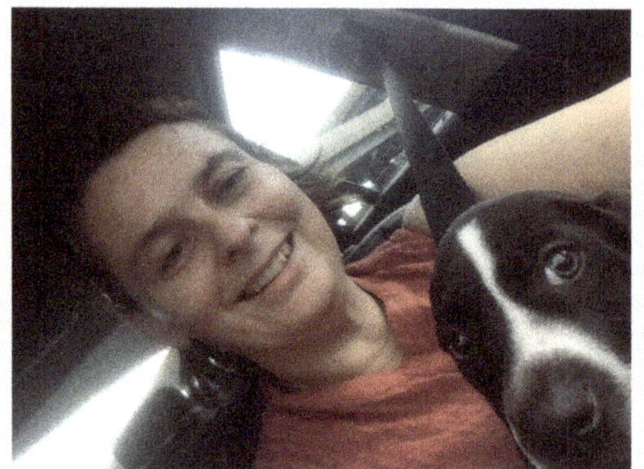
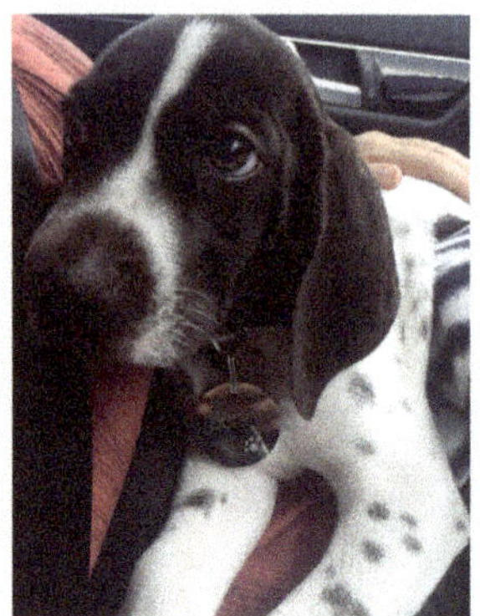

Baby Benni - the promise of a future

with excitement. A lady walked over to me and handed me this small, soft little bundle of joy. I buried my nose in her fur to inhale the sweet puppy smell and quietly whispered "Hello, Benni, I'm your mummy."

I quietly made a promise to baby Benni that if she took care of me and helped me through this terrible time, I would always be there for her.

It very quickly became clear why the training organisation at the time had recommended not having another dog while training my assistance dog (though this is something I no longer believe to be true). Rizzo disliked Benni and snapped at her every time she came close. Despite my best efforts, I would have to ask family to take Rizzo. Unfortunately, everyone already owned dogs or couldn't take her, so I cast my search wider and found someone who would make sure she had a loving home and keep me updated for a while to ensure she was settling in well.

I felt so much guilt over rehoming Rizzo and cried inconsolably all the way to and from dropping her off. This was an extremely difficult decision, but Rizzo settled in well to her new home, and I could focus on training my new puppy, even though I had no clue what I was doing! It's easy for people to judge from the outside, but I still believe rehoming a dog for their welfare is more humane and less selfish than keeping them just so you don't feel guilty or to keep up appearances.

Within a month of Benni coming home, Mum also got her puppy, Bella, and we started the training process together from afar. I was still struggling with PTSD symptoms, particularly with sleep disturbance, nightmares, severe anxiety, flashbacks and ongoing depression related to my current circumstances. Sleep was almost non-existent. Every tiny noise would wake me in a fright, my heart racing and brain always thinking the worst. My dreams were filled with failed resuscitations where I was responsible for someone's death and bleeding I just couldn't control. Every time I shut my eyes, I saw blood everywhere. In one of the recurring dreams, I was responsible for a large steel vat full of blood. There was a pipe running in and it kept overflowing onto the floor. I couldn't keep up with the flow of blood and all my attempts to turn off the valve failed.

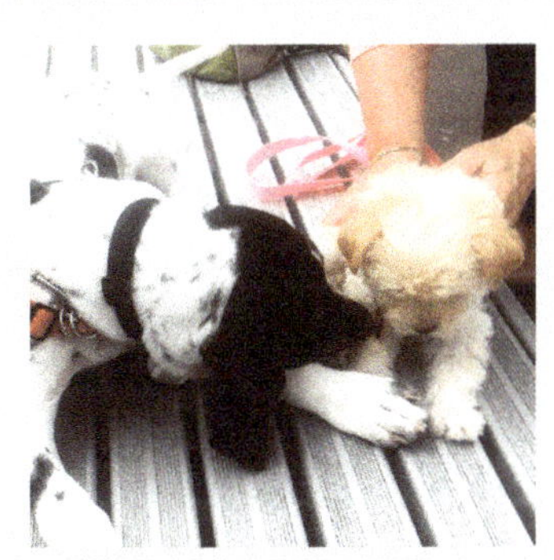

When Benni met Bella

Anxiety was at an all-time high, so I was jumping at shadows every time I moved. I had even lost my ability to reverse the car, anxiety overcoming me as soon as I tried, hands trembling and heart racing. I would eventually give up any attempt to leave the house. All this, of course, fed into the depression and growing sense of hopelessness. However, now every time I woke in a fright, startled with anxiety or trembled in fear, beside me was the beautiful Miss

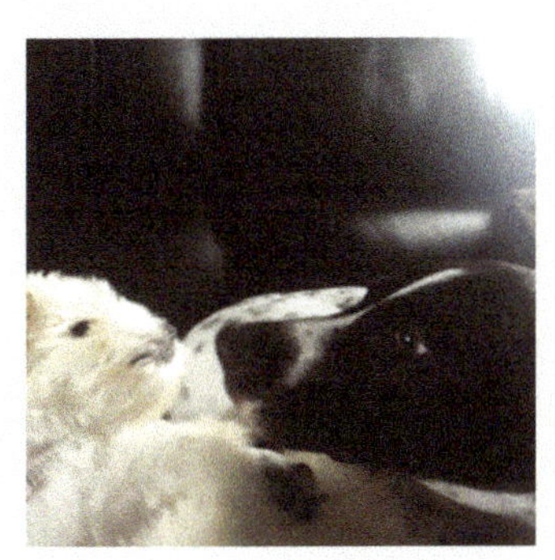

The start of a beautiful friendship

Benni with her warm, wet nose and innocent eyes. Her presence alone provided much-needed reassurance.

There was still a lot going on. My financial circumstances had deteriorated to the point where I was seriously considering declaring bankruptcy. I was on a sinking ship and bailing frantically without any impact. I was so terrified of bankruptcy I would have done absolutely anything to avoid it. Mum always instilled in me the idea of resourcefulness in difficult times, and this time was no different. When I was admitted to Healing House, Mum advised it would be wise to stock up on nonperishable food items, essential staples like toilet paper, cleaning products and dog essentials. She said it would help me to create some stability when everything else felt uncertain. My house started to look a little bit like the apocalypse was coming and I guess it probably was. I was still talking to creditors and trying to refinance. I desperately tried everything I possibly could to prevent bankruptcy but this was one of those times when Chicken Little was right – the sky really was falling in and my job now was just to survive it.

It's funny because nobody tells you what it's going to feel like when the rug is pulled out from underneath you and everything around you is taken away. From my perspective, I hadn't just lost my ability to function at work. It felt like I had lost my role as a doctor altogether, along with my decades-long relationship and financial security. I wasn't just falling apart or coming undone; I was being ripped apart piece by piece and I felt like there would be almost nothing left by the time it was over.

Once it became obvious I could no longer service my debts and my attempts to refinance were going to be unsuccessful, I finally took the plunge and, with a lot of tears and dread, declared bankruptcy. There's a lot of shame around this I have now overcome. Sometimes it's truly the only option and for me, at the time, it just had to be done. I was given a whole lot of paperwork to fill out and so began the horrible journey that would last exactly three years and one day.

I distinctly remember when they came to repossess my car. I thought I'd be more upset about the repossession of the Mercedes, but all I felt was relief as they put it onto the trailer and drove it away. The angst was over. The worst had happened. I was bankrupt, in more than one area of my life. The person that I dedicated so much time and energy becoming no longer existed and I began to mourn her loss.

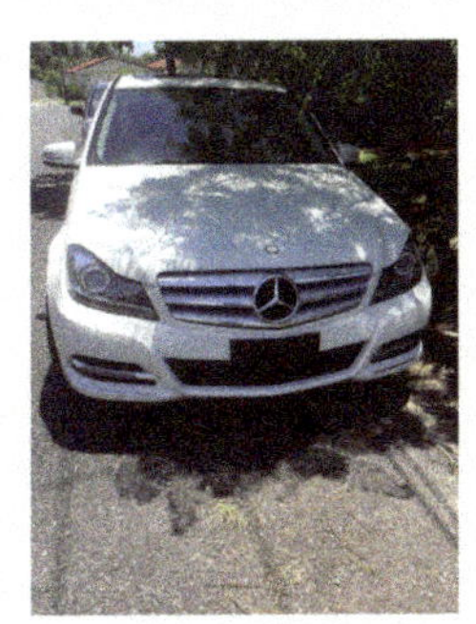

The Mercedes waiting to be repossessed

I realised I would need a car of some sort and reached out to my dad, knowing he always had a cheap car or two lying around. I talked to Dad and Nang, who were living on Russell Island at the time. Dad said he could help me with a little Mazda sedan with low kilometres, but I would have to get it on the road myself. He was happy to let me use it as it only cost him $300 at the time. I took my baby Benni with me and we headed to Russell Island. The car was perfect. It would require some mechanical repairs but I could live off my apocalyptic supplies for a couple of weeks so I could afford to fix it. Thank goodness for Mum and her resourceful advice, and thank goodness for Dad and his cars!

While staying with Dad, I had a lengthy discussion with him about my PTSD. Much to my surprise, he was vaguely interested and seemed to have a very good understanding of the symptoms. Eventually he talked about how he believed he also had PTSD from his time in prison and the challenge of reinventing himself after he got out. He talked about some of the terrible things he said he witnessed in prison, including gang rapes and torture, and spoke about how he survived by purposefully getting in trouble so he would be thrown in solitary confinement. He alluded to other horrible things he had to do to survive in prison but wouldn't elaborate. He shared how the nightmares never went away but how he just accepts them as part of life. Despite his mother holding the Bible and her faith close, Dad opened up about how he had a Bible brought to him in prison, but he could not make sense of a higher power in such a horrible world.

I really didn't expect such a frank conversation. Mum and Dad seemed to understand hardship and how to survive it better than most, but Dad had never shown an ounce of compassion or understanding for me, so this was a first. This discussion gave me amazing insight into what shaped Dad as a young man. How awful it must have been to survive in the prison system not long after losing his mum and how challenging it was to start again once released. This also gave me some hope that one day, maybe, I would be able to come back from all of this. I gratefully left with both the car and a greater understanding and empathy for my father. I completed all the little mechanical jobs and got it on the road. I was mobile again!

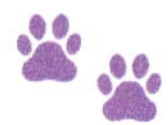

The unspoken truth about bankruptcy? There are a whole lot of minor consequences that can have a massive impact on your life. One of these was an inability to get a rental property to live in on my own. My lease was coming up for renewal. I couldn't afford the lease on my own but I also knew I wouldn't be able to get another rental on my own either. I couldn't work, so there was no regular work-related income and my credit rating was non-existent. I discussed this with my psychiatrist at the time and their advice was to talk to family to see if anyone could help. I spent so much of my life fiercely independent and strong; it was so hard to be vulnerable. I also tried so hard to be a good mum and, despite how loving and supportive they were, I still felt like a terrible burden on my children at this time. The psychiatrist reminded me that he believed as adults, any child would want their mum to have secure housing and get well. But I felt very disempowered as a mother having to ask my children for help.

I was very grateful when my son helped me to secure housing for six months, giving me valuable time to sort out what to do next. I wasn't the best version of myself at this time. I was having extreme difficulty with sleep, my mood was persistently low, I was irritable at best and generally not pleasant to be around.

The stress related to the management of bankruptcy was making my PTSD symptoms worse. Perhaps the most difficult thing to deal with at this time was the sense that my mind was failing me. For a very long time I had been functioning at a high level and relied on my brain and its ability to process things quickly to do so. I was suddenly unable to read a simple paragraph without feeling tired, could not process new information or apply critical thinking to new situations. I found it difficult to manage any task that might be even slightly challenging, even something as simple as parking a car straight. Training Benni was the only positive task I had to do each day and this kept me alive. If I stopped and spent any time dwelling on the negativity of the situation I was in, I simply would not have survived.

When she came home, I made a promise to this beautiful little puppy that if she took care of me through this extremely difficult time, I would always be there for her. This was a big job for such a tiny puppy, but she seemed to take it all in her stride and rose to the challenge every day with her unconditional love, innocence, cheeky disposition and willingness to learn. I felt useful because I needed to look after this beautiful puppy's needs and try to train her for her important job at the same time. I forged ahead, learning everything I possibly could about training an assistance animal and the techniques used to teach them complex tasks. I found reading extremely frustrating, so most of my learning was done through watching videos. I taught her how to go to the toilet on command and started trying to teach her how to walk politely on a leash.

Benni taught me how to speak some dog. It was fascinating to learn how dogs can also say "No" at times and, if you listened to them, you could communicate on an ever-deeper level. I was focused on the task. The recurrent small wins I was experiencing with her training were not only building positive momentum but also allowed me some relief from the constant miserable thoughts in my brain and the external circumstances that confirmed them.

Benni was spirited and had a mind of her own, behavioural traits I knew were required for assistance dogs, but also made training an enormous challenge at times. She repeatedly licked toads and ended up at the vet for intoxications. But she would also sit with me through my lost days, following my lead and not even getting up to go to the toilet unless I did. If I was sick, she would stay by my side and follow me around everywhere. If I was just in a funk and feeling sorry for myself, she would do something silly. I would come to learn she would misbehave when my mood was low, creating a much-needed distraction.

One of her favourite things to do as a puppy was to steal items and wait for the chase. One day I was really struggling with low mood. I was moping around the house, getting ready to take a shower, feeling sad and sorry for myself. I watched as she stealthily walked past me into the bedroom, stole the underwear I'd laid out for after my shower (thankfully, it was clean), and proceeded to dash out past me and into the yard as I chased close behind. I was initially really annoyed as I scurried out into the yard after her without any shoes on, half-dressed and limping after treading on several prickles, yelling, "Benni, *stop*!" several times to no avail.

Then I watched as she deliberately looked out the corner of her eye and, with an almost cheeky grin, she catapulted my underwear high into the sky like a beachball at a concert. As I drew closer, while still giving me the side-eye, she picked them up again and threw them with glee back into the air. By that stage I was in hysterics. After much frivolity chasing Benni with my undies in her mouth in the yard, I finally got them back and headed inside to have my shower, giggling under my breath, "Bloody dog."

I realised this was the first time I felt joy in a long time. I didn't know it yet, but she was doing her job beautifully. During the worst time in my life, this little puppy did what no human could – she made me laugh!

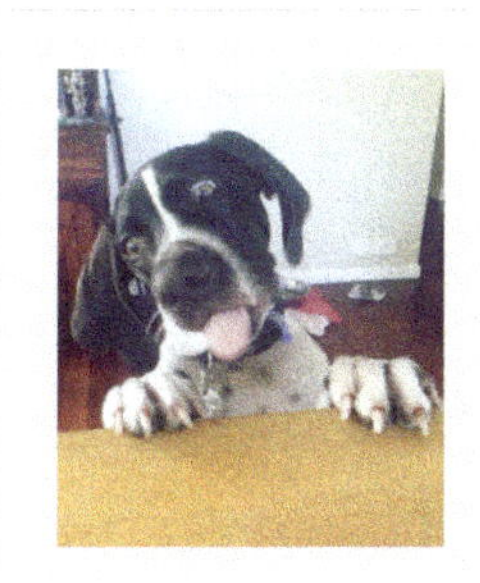

Crazy eye

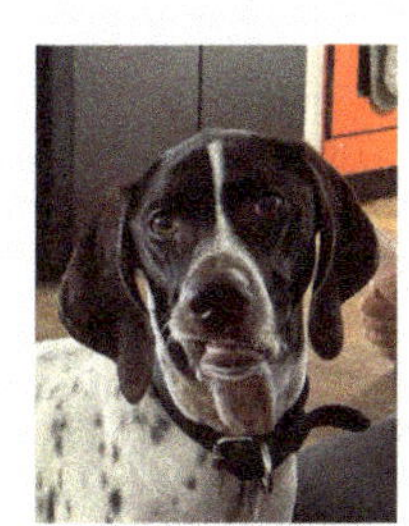

Contemplating mischief

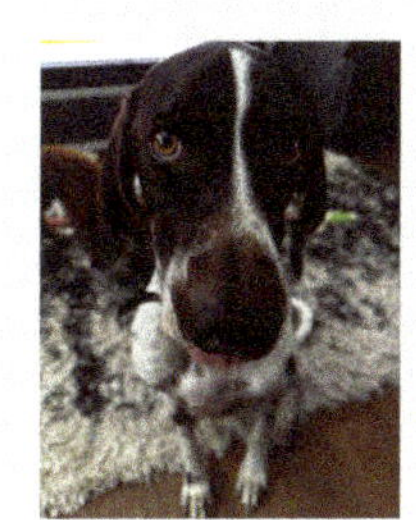

It wasn't me!

During her first year of life, Benni was trained to provide emotional support, to wake me up from nightmares and to disrupt unhelpful behaviours. I had developed a condition called chronic idiopathic urticaria. This is where you have a prolonged period with daily eruptions of hives (itchy lumps usually associated with allergy) without any known cause. The hives were unbearable, especially at night, when they disrupted my sleep. I was constantly scratching and developed some areas called plaques. This is where the hives all come together and the whole area swells. I was taking all sorts of medicines for this and applying topical steroids a few times a day just to manage the discomfort. One of the problems with this condition is when you scratch, more substances are released that increase the urge to scratch.

I set about training Benni to stop me from scratching. She was absolutely brilliant at this task and took her job very seriously. If I started to scratch, Benni would nudge my hand away with her nose gently. If I kept going, she would become more forceful with her nose. If I still wasn't listening, she would use her paw to push my hand away. In assistance dog training, this is called an escalation protocol. She refused to let me scratch at all and gradually the angry skin around the plaques settled down. With Benni's support, after eight months of daily discomfort, it was finally bearable. It made me appreciate her so much more.

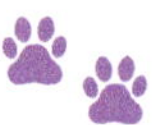

The lease was once again coming up for renewal and, not wanting to impose on my children anymore, I talked to Mum about getting a rental together. Without her, I was facing the real possibility of having no home at all. Thankfully, she agreed and we found an amazing house, with dual living capacity, to rent on the water in Golden Beach on the Sunshine Coast.

This house was a bit rundown, but the location was outstanding and it even had a swimming pool! We put in a joint application and, because Mum had such a great credit rating at the time, they approved our application despite my financial situation. We couldn't believe it! In late 2017, we moved into our house near the beach, Mum living downstairs with Bella, Benni and I living upstairs. I was a little worried about living with Mum as we were in a wonderful place in our relationship and I didn't want to ruin it. I was still in such a difficult situation and there was a long road of recovery ahead of me, but Mum said she was all in. It was so much better not to feel like I was burdening the children and this would be a fresh start for both Mum and me.

When you're unwell with an invisible illness, you're often met with a degree of suspicion, as if you're feigning or exaggerating your symptoms. I found this very hard to take and it wasn't just "the system" that made you feel this way. The stigma around mental health is real and I was starting to experience this unpleasant phenomenon. Some, it seemed, wouldn't even let the term "PTSD" pass their lips, often professing to know more than the forensic psychiatrists and countless psychometric diagnostic tests (standardised, objective measurements of mental attributes including personality) I would end up undergoing.

This disbelief remains one of the hardest parts of this whole journey to take. I couldn't believe people who knew me seemed to prefer to believe either I was faking it or I had some far more significant (in their eyes) psychiatric problem such as bipolar, schizophrenia or a personality disorder. This really added to the trauma I was experiencing. I was initially quite frightened of the forensic psychiatric assessments, thinking that there might be something fundamentally wrong with me, just as my father had made me believe so long ago. It's quite intimidating having your whole personality probed.

However, despite how difficult these examinations were, I'm now extremely grateful I went through them. It doesn't seem to stop people accusing me of being "crazy" despite the real experts independently finding no evidence to support those claims. This knowledge has quietened my mind and stopped me from believing those unhelpful couch experts. I now generally understand these accusations come from a place of anger in the individual and have nothing to do with me or my mental health.

The stigma I experienced also extended to medical professionals. It's confronting to see how readily physical symptoms are sometimes dismissed once you have a mental health diagnosis. There is a whole group of online forums dedicated to supporting people who have experienced what they refer to as medical gaslighting. As a doctor, I witnessed times when I felt the preconceived ideas of medical professionals impacted on their attitudes towards patients with mental health diagnoses. I always disliked this and refused to see people as their label.

I have observed that if you have a broken bone people have sympathy for you, but when you have a mental health diagnosis people seem suspicious of you. We like to think we've come a long way as a society but I believe this is mostly rhetoric. In my opinion, mental health stigma is rife even within the halls of medicine and it's an awful thing to experience when you're at your most vulnerable.

Even if I did have some other mental health issue or personality disorder, why would that make me a worse person in the eyes of others? Isn't that the very definition of stigma? Perhaps it just makes it easier for others to justify how they choose to see or label you. I will forever be thankful for the awful process of recurrent forensic examinations as it has made me understand myself better and stops the internal critic from hurting me any more than it already has.

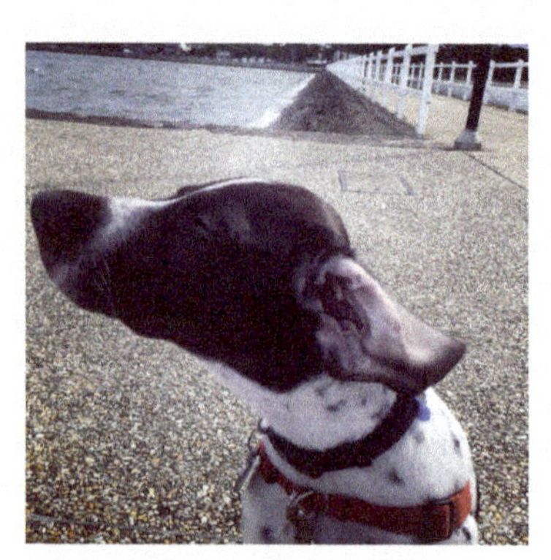

"I love the wind in my ears"

Through all these times, Benni was always there with a gentle nudge and soft fur. I have a saying: "Thank God for the dog." Whenever I experienced this sort of stigma, I would say this over and over in my head to help me get through it. Benni never passed judgement. I knew she loved me and that wasn't dependent on how well or sick I was. She didn't care what my diagnosis was, if I was in a good or bad mood, how much money I earnt or what my profession was. She just loved me exactly as I was. Every time I came through the door, she would happily greet me like I was the best thing in her day, cuddle me and lean her head on my leg, pressing down heavily to show how connected she was. This kind of unconditional love was restorative. This is what got me through these difficult times.

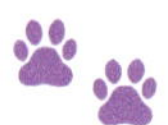

Living in this huge house on the water with Mum was lovely. We would take the dogs over the road to what we affectionately referred to as "Benni's beach". Benni would ask to go there three times a day and absolutely loved swimming in the water. Her training was still a huge challenge with problems like reactivity (barking at dogs and people) and terrible pulling while on her lead, adding to the toad licking and stealing of underwear. She was still very much a work in progress.

We found some good trainers, but many were too far away or too expensive. We eventually started with an organisation that certified assistance dogs but they were cautioning me about what they called "red flags" in Benni that may prevent her from qualifying. I was someone with a severe anxiety disorder, so saying my dog had "red flags" and implying that she may not make it as an assistance dog, was devastating to me. My anxieties grew and continued to impact on her training. I was really surprised by this language, and what I felt represented a lack of understanding around how this would affect me. The trainer provided me with several strategies but our issues persisted. I tried several different trainers, lots of different strategies but her behavioural issues remained unchanged. I struggled to find approaches that I felt were effective for Benni. Naturally, I saw this as a challenge and set about learning everything I could about the dog training methods I was being told to use.

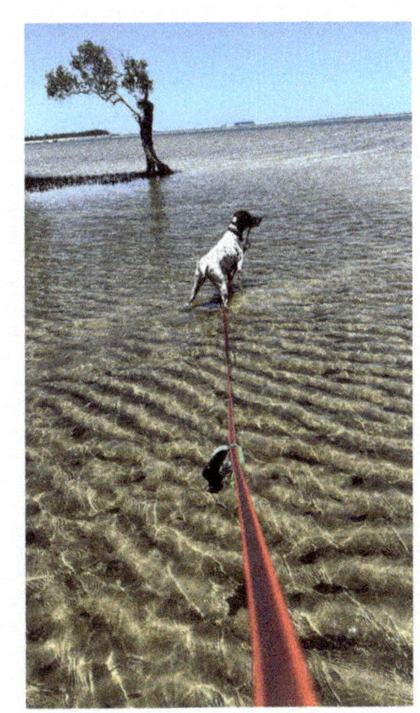

Enjoying "Benni's beach"

I was out with one of these dog trainers one day and, while I wasn't aware of what she was doing at the time, I now understand this approach to be a technique referred to as "flooding". Flooding is where you expose an animal (Benni in this case) to a feared stimulus (a weird surface in the local waterfront park) in the hope that their anxiety will reduce over time. She took Benni to a walkway with a strange surface and Benni stopped dead in her tracks, pulling back hard on the collar and lead. The trainer started trying to move her forward by gently pulling on the lead, just as I was saying, "I don't think that will work with Benni."

Suddenly, like soap through wet hands, Benni slipped the collar and ran for her little life in the opposite direction. She was playing the "chase me" game we had played so many times with my underwear. Mostly she was trying to get away from the scary surface. Benni ran along the foreshore park and straight to the beach, her ears flapping in the breeze. I was grateful at this point she didn't go on the road on the other side of the park. We were right next to a set of lights so traffic was slow, but it was still a concern.

We both chased her, but she continued to evade us as people watched the comical commotion unfolding before them. Unfortunately, she made the awful decision to come back up towards the park and dart across the road. There was nothing I wouldn't do for this dog and apparently that now included running in front of traffic. I found myself standing in front of a big Mack truck, with my feeble hands waving frantically in the air in an attempt to stop the driver from running over Benni. He slowed down just enough for Benni to run back in front of him and into the bushes in the park, thankfully also giving me enough time to avoid being hit by the truck. As I reached the edge of the park, she finally allowed me to approach and I was able to grab her by the scruff of the neck as the trainer made her way back with Benni's collar and lead. I hugged her with all my might, so relieved that my baby Benni was okay.

"Mummy's got you, Benni. I'm so sorry."

Exhausted by the chase, we went back up to the car to cut the training session short. While we were debriefing, I safely tucked Benni away in the car and promptly oozed to the ground, leaning up against the car. I was hyperventilating, dizzy, short of breath and had chest pain.

I was aware of the trainer's voice, asking, "Jodi, are you okay? Do I need to call an ambulance?" But I couldn't respond properly.

I gasped and quickly got out, "Just. Wait." I knew this was a panic attack, so I started to control my breathing. Gradually the chest pain and shortness of breath settled, and I was able to tell the trainer I was okay. I was too embarrassed to tell her I'd had a panic attack. Instead, we agreed that maybe I was getting sick. After this experience, I no longer believed the trainer knew better than me how to handle my dog. I started looking for a new organisation but resolved to do most of the training myself and trust my own judgement from then on.

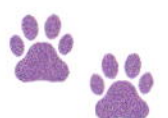

I started helping Mum to train Bella. I was becoming a bit of an expert and wanted to share this with Mum. We worked together with Bella and Benni and finally started with a new organisation. They seemed to have a good understanding of the anxiety associated with PTSD as well as positive training techniques. They also relied on you to do much of your dog's training yourself, which was just fine with me. When Benni met the head of the new organisation, she was feeding off my anxiety and was reactive, barking at him and the other dogs. Instead of talking about red flags, he reassured us that we could address this issue and that the more relaxed I was, the more relaxed she would be. I had to fake it until I made it. My newfound confidence in training techniques worked beautifully, and Benni's reactivity started to reduce and gradually disappeared.

We were finally getting somewhere and could do some training in public. I had become somewhat of a hermit so it was hard to get out of the house at first. I started to see that training the dog was beneficial to the human as well. Having to pretend I wasn't anxious to leave the house helped Benni with her anxiety. Over time, I became more confident getting out and about and I began to think we were going to make it as an assistance dog team!

My life challenges were ticking away in the background and recurrently created stressful situations. There were ongoing treatment schedules and reporting requirements for bankruptcy and I was also organising my divorce. I'm still amazed I got through all of it. Benni, with her entertaining antics and ongoing training requirements, kept me going. When we went out for her twice daily short training sessions, her ongoing behavioural challenges kept my mind active looking for solutions. She was a source of joy and I was absolutely enamoured with this cheeky, furry little creature. She was just as loving towards me.

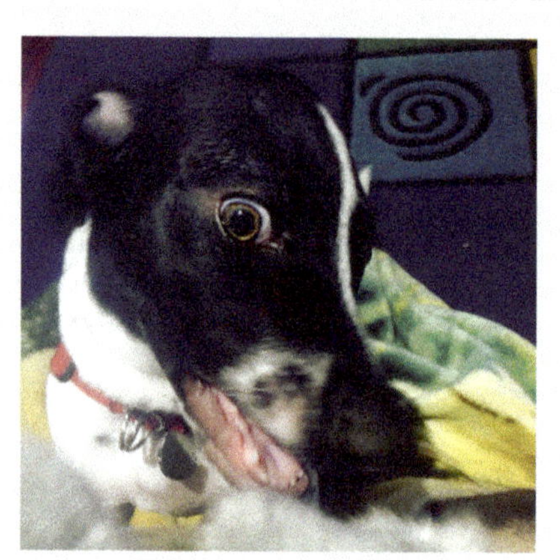
My cheeky little puppy

Towards the end of my time in this house, Eliot married his beautiful partner and, with support, I was able to attend the wedding. I'm grateful we could all come together to celebrate before they left to live overseas. I was very upset because I knew my finances would prevent me from visiting them. Another unintended consequence of bankruptcy is you can't go overseas without permission; you effectively relinquish your passport until bankruptcy is over. I cried so much as I saw them off.

Near the end of the lease on this house, I received a small payout for my neck injury and reached a point where I was able to make a Total and Permanent Disability (TPD) claim on my superannuation. In general, I understood that superannuation and insurance claims are protected money, so bankruptcy can't access them to recover your debt. I knew exactly what to do with the money. After getting legal clearance, I planned to buy a house so I would no longer have to worry about the roof over my head. I really wanted to do something to thank Mum for her support and helped her to find and purchase a little cabin at the caravan park in Golden Beach. I felt so proud to have been able to help

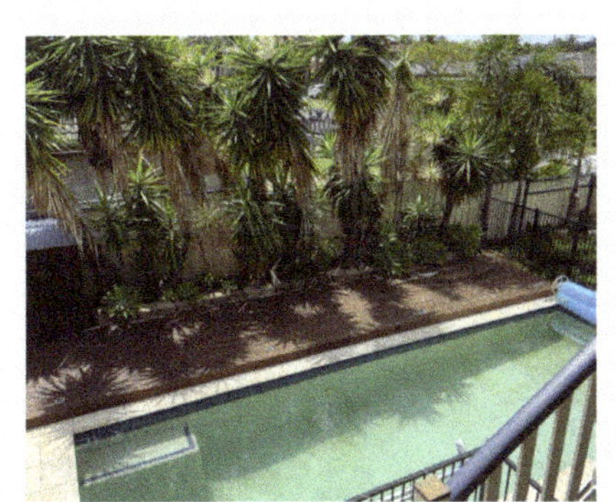

Overlooking the pool of my very first house

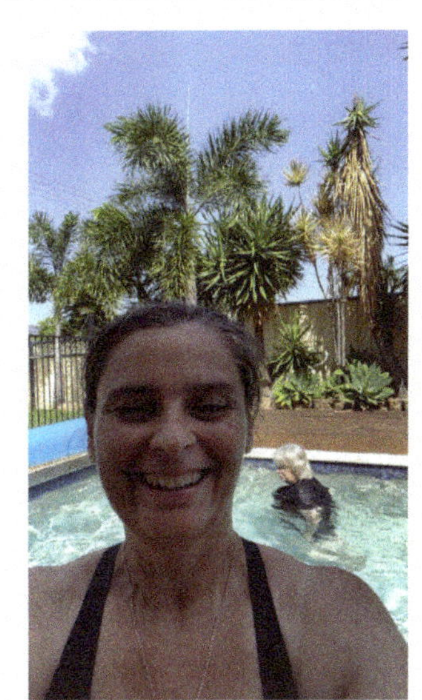

Mum enjoying the pool

her get a little home she could call her own. She did most of the work to renovate this little cabin with a bit of help from family.

For the first time in my life, I also owned my own home. I bought a lovely, two-storey house with a pool, near the water in a little outer suburb of Brisbane. No-one could take this away from me. I finally had a tiny bit of security. After a lot of discussion, Angie agreed to move in with me.

While the children were growing up, I always tried to think of their needs and put them first. This time, while I framed it like I was being considerate, in hindsight I wasn't thinking about the needs of others at all. In all honesty, I was scared of living alone, of feeling isolated and uncertain of what life would be like without any of my family around.

Eliot was gone and Angie was my beautiful baby girl, I didn't want to lose her. Among all of this, I was still struggling with a complete lack of self-esteem and lost the confidence to look after myself. My sense of identity had evaporated in almost all respects except for my role as a mum, so I was going to hold on to this tightly.

SAVED BY A DOG

When we met, my day had turned into night
Your soft fur and wet nose touched my soul, I knew they were right
I would be saved by a dog
Your presence created chaos and joy where there had been only sorrow
With you I felt like I had a future, there was hope for a tomorrow
All the treatments in the world could not compare
To the love I felt whenever you were there
Endless training, equipment and walks
Beat every medication, no need for long talks
You gave life back its meaning and purpose
With you by my side nothing could hurt us
We achieved together what I thought was out of reach
Your unconditional love and support, so much you had to teach
As you age and your body grows weary, my dear friend
My heart and soul will be with you to the very end
I will find you over the rainbow bridge, I will bring a long chew
Because I was saved by a dog as special as you

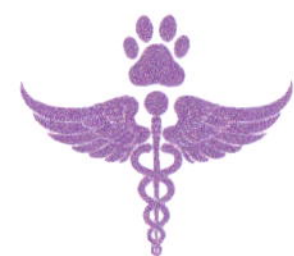

Mum settled into her new little home and so had we. Benni's training was going very well, and both she and Bella were on track to pass their Public Access Test (PAT). This is a test to confirm that the team can work safely in public and the dog meets the standards of behaviour and hygiene required. We were getting ready to sit the PAT when one night everything changed.

I was used to Benni waking me up as she was trained to rouse me from nightmares. This night was different. She abruptly jumped off the bed onto the floor, immediately vomiting, which woke me up. I got up and turned the light on to offer reassurance, thinking she must have eaten something she shouldn't have.

She was still vomiting and wasn't taking a breath in between. Staring directly at me as if asking for help, her mouth was open and her face was scrunched up like she was in pain. A large chunk of a treat eaten earlier in the day plopped onto the floor and then she stopped breathing. I started yelling out to Angelina to come and help. *She's choking to death and there's nothing I can do. I can't lose her!* I checked her airway as she stiffened and slipped out of my arms onto the floor. Her teeth were visible and she still wasn't breathing, but there was no obstruction to her airway. She started convulsing.

"Benni, no!"

I screamed as I cleared anything that may cause her injury and kept her head from hitting the leg of the bed. Her legs started to move back and forth on the floor as if she was paddling in the water, but she was no longer conscious. My medical training kicked in and I realised this was a familiar pattern to me. She wasn't choking at all – she was having a grand mal (generalised) seizure. After several minutes, the seizure finally stopped and she began to breathe. She was disoriented and couldn't walk properly. I scooped her up, carried her down the stairs and put her in the car, all the time reassuring her, "Mummy's got you. Mummy's got you."

Angie drove and I stayed in the back with Benni, calling the vet on the way. She was sleepy and disoriented for the whole drive. When we arrived, I told the vet how important she was, "This isn't just any dog – she's an assistance dog."

I conveyed how much I absolutely loved this dog, pleading, "I need her to be okay." The vet assessed her and finally came out, "She's recovering from a seizure. We can't be sure what caused it but I would like to keep her in overnight for observation."

I agreed and was then faced with a special dilemma for the first of many times. I was asked to pay a huge deposit and make decisions based on cost about her care. Living in a country with a publicly funded healthcare system, I was used to decisions being made based on clinical need, not cost. But this was veterinary medicine, not human medicine. It immediately occurred to me that if I didn't have the money left over from the purchase of the house, that night I may have found myself having to decide between money and her care, potentially her survival. I never wanted to be in that position again.

Benni went on to have a horrible two weeks, with readmissions and expensive investigations into why she had this seizure. No cause was found and the vet advised that if she didn't have another seizure in six months this may have been a one-off. I crossed my fingers and hoped that would be the case. I also started a Benni Fund so I would be prepared if it happened again. After six months seizure free, Benni and Bella sat their PAT and passed with flying colours. We made it – we were an accredited, working assistance dog team. It was a very proud moment.

Not long after passing her PAT, Benni had another seizure, was required to stop her public access work and was diagnosed with epilepsy. It would take trialling many different drug combinations over months to get her stable again.

We were meant to find each other. Benni was able to support me through many difficult times in my life and I had the knowledge to manage her seizure disorder, administer prescribed emergency medications and take care of her when she was sick. With each new medication, Benni would lose control of her back legs, be confused and sleepy, and require physical support with mobilising to the toilet. It was breaking my heart to see her suffer so much but the vet reassured me that we would get the right balance eventually. She spent years helping me through difficult times and now it was my turn to help her, just as I had promised the day I brought her home.

Apart from Benni's health challenges, living in this little house was an absolute pleasure. After spending a lifetime renting, I had no concept of what it was like to own my own house. If I wanted to attach something to the wall, I didn't need anyone's permission. Conversely, if I did any damage, it was all my responsibility. Looking after this house was all up to me.

The unravelling was complete. I felt like I was unemployable, could no longer use any of my qualifications to earn a living, and with my divorce finalised, Covid-19 hit the world. It seemed like the sky really was falling. On the upside, I had continued my practice of having apocalyptic supplies, hardly ever left the house, and therefore there was no-one to go and visit, so the impact was minimal for me compared to some. The state of the world made me think carefully about the future. I was acutely aware that any money I had wasn't going to last and I would quickly be in trouble if I didn't plan and start retraining towards something new. It was time to rebuild what was left of my life. It was time to go out on my own and survive in this new world by myself.

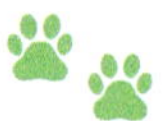

The journey back to functionality began with a very simple online course in animal nutrition and massage, which I started but never finished. The reading and learning were very difficult for my brain. While it was demoralising, it was clear that the more I used my brain, the more it would recover. Eventually, I enrolled in a dog grooming course, with more hands-on and less reading requirements. Could this be my new direction? I loved dogs and Miss Benni could always be with me, even if I was working or she was sick. I asked for special consideration for the online learning components I knew I would have difficulty with and this really helped me to get my brain working again without too much pressure. I was so excited when I passed. This new sense of self-efficacy gave me the confidence to plan my next move.

I bought a second little house with the rest of the protected money, and Benni and I made the big move to live on the Sunshine Coast to begin rebuilding our lives and to be closer to Mum as she got older. I was finally discharged from bankruptcy and decided to create a little grooming salon and dog training business in my new home, while continuing to train assistance dogs for other people like me. I was excited, ready to start again. Life had been on hold for long enough.

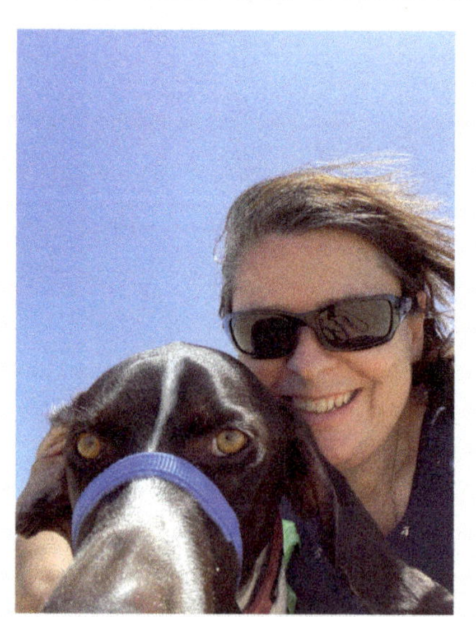

Happy times with Benni

This house was on a main road so it was a bit of a compromise, an investment that was a stepping stone to the end goal. I hoped the property would appreciate enough to allow me to buy a house near the beach on the Sunshine Coast, the ultimate goal for retirement. The grooming salon was a raging success, but I really didn't enjoy the work. While working with dogs was a pleasure, I found forcing them to be groomed when they didn't enjoy it was truly awful. There were other courses I enrolled in, but the stress of assessments and readings led me to pull out. It was going to take a while longer before my brain would be recovered enough to do another course. If a task was difficult, I just had to stop, or I would get extremely frustrated with myself and then feel demoralised.

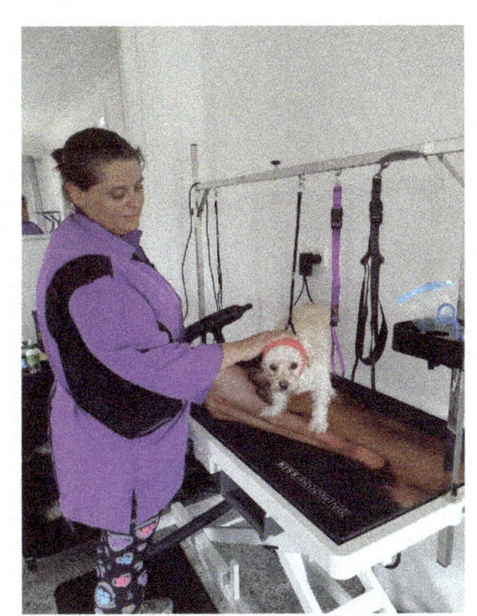

Grooming salon - Bella hated the drier

I worked daily on improving my reading ability and tried to build my tolerance to frustration. Working with dogs was clearly helping. What I really wanted to focus on was dog training but I couldn't find anyone with an appropriate course I could complete that was also in line with my focus on ethical methods. Benni changed the way I see dogs forever. These beautiful sentient beings have a whole language of their own and I felt training them should involve a mutual learning of communication. I also felt strongly that they should be able to give or remove consent and, in my opinion, deserved to be treated with gentle kindness and compassion. This is the way Benni always treated me.

There's good evidence that trauma and PTSD can impact on the brain's ability to function.[3] I was relying a lot on Benni for emotional support but also on others for help with the things that caused me the most frustration that my brain just wouldn't do. These were mostly tech-related issues, which I had a problem with at the best of times. Having only learnt to turn on a computer at age 24, I wasn't very tech savvy and learning anything to do with tech was more than my damaged brain could handle.

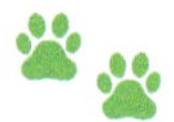

Benni had been doing well until one day she endured a long seizure followed by two short seizures in the car on the way to the vet. The seizures stopped on their own, but she was still admitted. This was a nightmare in the two-storey house. I hurt my back getting her to the car, forgot the child lock, and she thrashed in the car on the way, making it dangerous for us both. After she came home, I would have to support most of her weight going up and down the stairs every time she needed to use the toilet. I quickly realised that I would need a low-set house both for myself as I aged but also for Benni's safety. We would only end up staying a year in this house before closing the salon, selling up everything I owned, and looking for the dream house by the beach. It was a necessary move that came with its blessings and curses.

Unintended consequences had been a feature of this whole period of my life, and I was unaware of how my choices and behaviours were impacting on others at the time. I made many mistakes that I only understand now in hindsight. My behaviour and attitudes during my illness had not only caused hurt but also contributed to difficulties in many of my relationships. My choice that fateful day in 2014 when I overdosed on antidepressants had a flow-on effect that would affect my whole life. What I didn't appreciate at the time is how it would also impact on those around me.

I had lost every part of who I was since that horrible day and now I felt my role as a good mum slipping away. This loss would cut deeper than all the others. This was the one thing I thought I was good at – the turning point in my life and my greatest joy. I felt like I was failing in this role now! I feel I had gone from a successful, confident and self-assured provider for the whole family to completely obliterated, unable to work and with PTSD impacting on every aspect of my functionality. I appreciate that from the outside this must have been very difficult to watch. I leaned on others to share the grief and hardship during this time, something that felt necessary for survival. In my mind, the people around me had witnessed my decline and experienced the fallout of this difficult time. My children have always been so important to me. I love them more than I could ever express. I will always worry about any hurt my illness may have caused them; this is one thing I never intended and will always be deeply sorry for.

My thoughts went back to that day in 2014. *Would they have been better off if I had died?* I was struggling to keep myself together, but I knew I had to keep going. I was grieving all the perceived losses. Feeling incredibly isolated and alone, I reconnected with my amazing psychologist and focused back in on Benni and how we could start our new chapter together. *Thank God for the dog!* My psychologist is an amazing human being and I am forever grateful for her professionalism and support. She reminded me how important Benni was, how there had been many good years with the family, many good memories, "Focusing on what you have and your good memories can help." She has a way of helping me come to my own logical conclusions. We agreed that there were lots of great things happening in my life and focusing on these may help me to get through any grief I was feeling.

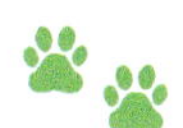

The market had miraculously boomed at just the right time. I found a little three-bedroom house to renovate, 300 metres from the beach, which I affectionately referred to as the "dog house". I was now only a few minutes' walk from Mum's place. Mum was expressing concern about my welfare as I was really struggling with the added loss of my role as a good mum and the significant guilt associated with the damage the past few years of illness and recovery had left in my wake. It was making me physically ill and there were days so dark I couldn't see the point in going on.

Mum was an enormous support during this time; her gentle and sometimes challenging voice of reason ever present. Whenever I struggled, Mum would remind me that making a mistake didn't make me a bad person and then redirect my attention back to Benni and whatever new project I had on the go at the time. Benni was my constant companion throughout all the hardship and she remained my main reason for getting out of bed in the morning. My daily internal mantra had become *Thank God for the dog.*

Dog training was my passion, and I continued to help people with disabilities train their dogs through a great relationship with a nearby training organisation. I started to notice something unexpected. People often commented that the process of training their dog felt therapeutic for them, not just for their dog. In fact, a passing comment during one of my dog training sessions sparked a new way of thinking that stayed with me. It planted the seed of an idea: that perhaps there was a way to combine my love of dog training with therapy and build something meaningful from that intersection.

The dream was still to become an accredited assistance dog trainer and build my own organisation, but this felt a bit out of reach as I couldn't find the appropriate course. *Perhaps I could retrain as a counsellor and include my animals in therapy.* I had experienced how therapeutic the relationship with an assistance dog can be, and Benni had taught me so much about training. While we renovated the house, this would have to take a back seat.

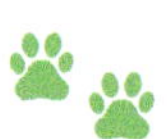

In February 2022, while living in one room, Benni, the builders and I gutted the little house and started the complete renovation to convert it into a five-bedroom, three-bathroom house with a pool. The perfect place to live and work until retirement. Mum came over frequently, overseeing all the work and providing her valuable insight into each decision.

The joy of this new stage in life would be short-lived. Not long after we started this renovation, Mum was experiencing vague abdominal pain and felt like she was getting recurrently dismissed by doctors. At my insistence, she finally went to a GP we both knew and trusted, and had a scan. She got a call the same day to come in to see the doctor and rang me to tell me she was returning in the afternoon. I knew this was an indication of bad news and I think she did too. I cancelled work, dropped everything and went with her. The news wasn't good. They discovered a mass on her ovary and some other changes consistent with ovarian cancer. The GP indicated she wouldn't know for sure until Mum had a biopsy, but it looked like cancer.

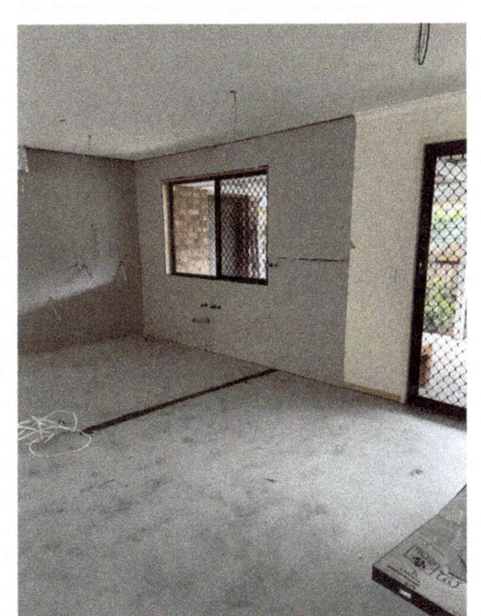

The "dog house" gutted and ready to renovate

While we were expecting bad news, we were still surprised. *Cancer? No-one in the family has had cancer.* Mum had been so healthy her whole life. She was in shock and really didn't know how to take the news. Mum was adamant she didn't want to tell anyone until she got a proper diagnosis. Sadly, the biopsy would confirm ovarian cancer with some involvement of the omentum (the little fatty flap that covers the abdominal organs). She was booked to have chemotherapy and then

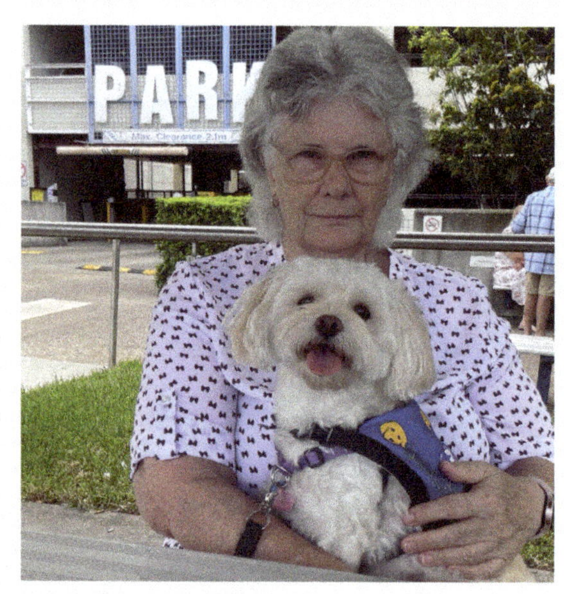

Bella doing her job waiting for the first oncology appointment

a clearance operation. On April 19, 2022, we met the oncology team at the Royal Women's Hospital in Brisbane. They confirmed what I already knew: the five-year survival rate for ovarian cancer was less than 30 per cent for people with cancer as advanced as hers looked, but they would wait for the operation to confirm this. Her first round of chemotherapy would occur before the operation and started on May 20.

I picked Mum up for her first round of chemo. She was visibly anxious and concerned. Bella had been up all night vomiting and she seemed to be in pain. She appeared okay at the time I picked Mum up, so we left some water and I reassured Mum that once she was settled at the hospital, I would come back to check on Bella. When I got back it was clear Bella had been vomiting again. She looked very unwell. I took her to the nearest vet where she was diagnosed with acute pancreatitis and admitted. There we were, Mum in hospital having chemo and poor Bella in hospital having treatment as well. What a shemozzle! Mum and

Bella were sick for the next few days but thankfully both were soon at home recovering.

Day six post chemo, Mum deteriorated with a fever. She called me after being in pain all day to tell me she had a temperature over 38 degrees. I advised her to call an ambulance and went over to stay with her until the ambulance arrived, taking Bella home with me. Mum was neutropenic, meaning her neutrophil count (the white blood cells needed to fight infection) was dangerously low. An impacted gallstone had also blocked off a tube called the common bile duct. The combination of fever and low neutrophils is a common but dangerous complication of chemotherapy called febrile neutropenia (fever with low immunity). Bella couldn't visit her, as she was still sick herself, so we got permission for Benni to visit Mum. She was in a lot of pain; the team were still trying to figure out her management plan while they stabilised her.

Benni was amazing. She hopped up on Mum's bed, gently placing her feet on the bed, careful not to hurt Mum. You could tell she understood how sick Mum was, intuitively knowing she needed to be gentle. Benni placed her head on Mum's thigh, allowing Mum to caress her head until

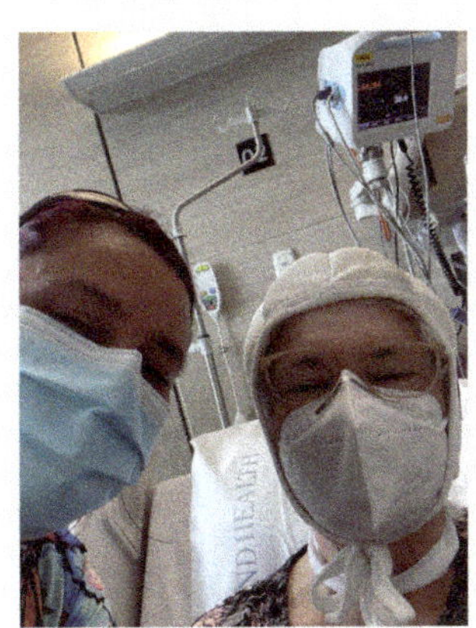

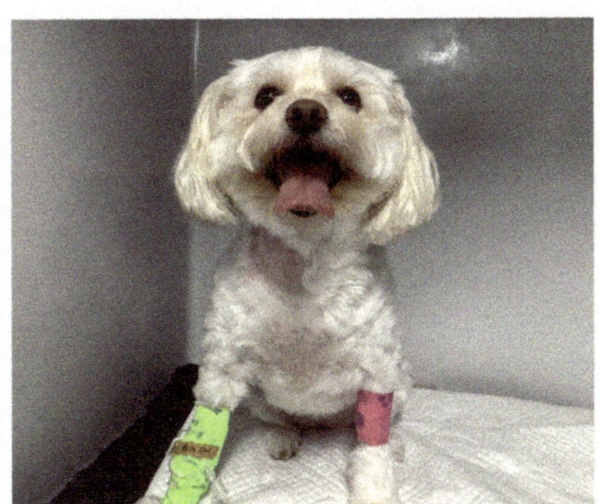

Round 1, day one of chemo with Mum and Bella in hospital

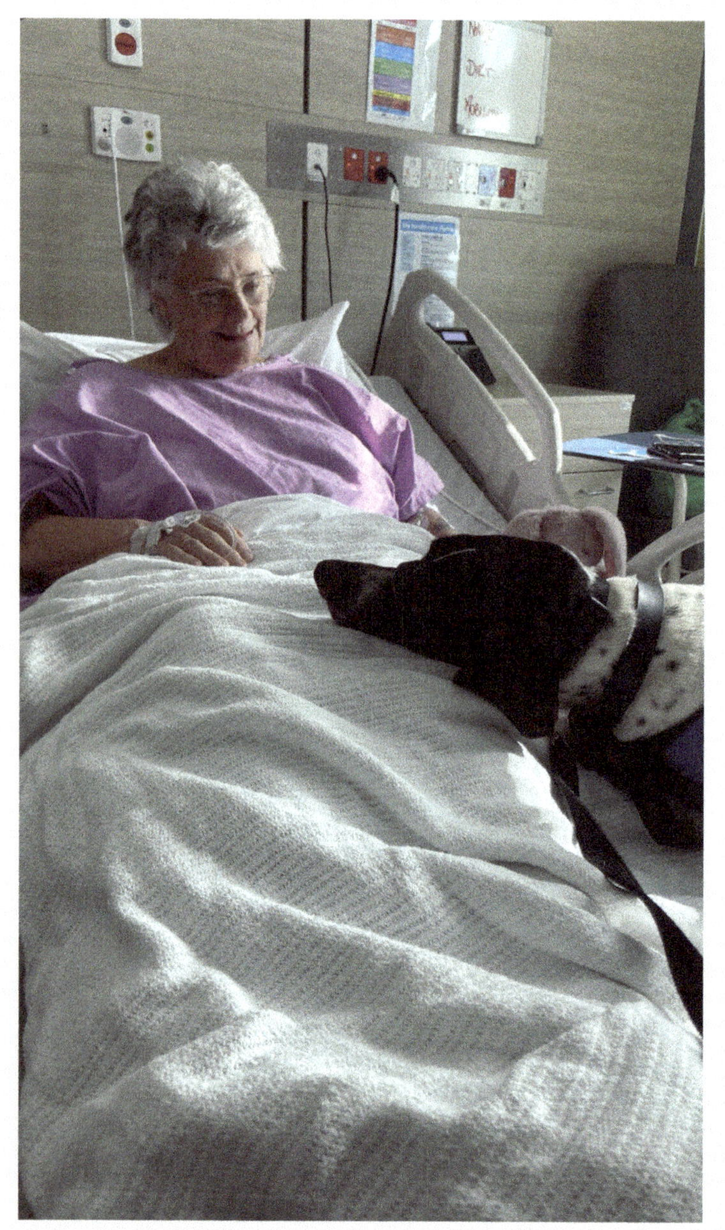

Benni visiting Mum when Bella was sick

she felt better. You could see the stress draining from Mum's body as she patted Benni and it warmed my heart. Mum provided this same support to Benni so many times before after her seizures, and in this incredibly vulnerable time Benni had the same compassion and care for Mum. This truly cemented in me the importance of sharing the amazing healing power of assistance dogs with others.

One night during this hospital admission I got a frantic, distressed call from Mum on the ward. She had been experiencing persistent pain for hours without any relief. I tried to reassure her, "Mum, press your call button again – they will come."

"They're so busy," she said through tears, the pain obvious in her voice. She agreed to press the button again but I could tell that she didn't want to ask for pain relief.

When I got off the phone, I knew Mum would be reluctant to advocate for herself. I flew into action. I collected Bella, who was much better, and we went to visit Mum. I didn't tell her I was coming – I knew she would tell me not to – but I also knew this is what she needed. As soon as we walked through the door Mum burst into tears and buried herself in Bella's fur with a big hug, sobbing about the pain. Bella listened intently to Mum's distress and showed she was just as happy to see her. It was amazing to see the instant calming effect that the mere presence of Bella had on Mum. I left her with Bella to talk to a member of staff who got Mum some pain relief. They were indeed very busy, but once I communicated the severity and duration of Mum's pain they recognised the urgency and responded promptly.

We waited until her pain was under control and I took Miss Bella home. The next morning when I came in to see her, Mum held my hand tightly and through tears said, "I wanted to tell you, Jo, what you did, bringing Bella in last night, was the most thoughtful thing anyone has ever done for me."

The pain relief was helpful but seeing Bella was just the medicine she needed. After trying conservative management and injections to increase her neutrophils they decided to do a procedure to remove the stone through the oesophagus (down your mouth). This worked and she finally started to improve. She reacted to the antibiotics and changing them would delay discharge. On June 4, after nine days in hospital, Mum finally got to come home. That was the first dose of the first round of chemotherapy, so we hoped it wasn't going to be like this every time!

Mum completed the rest of her chemotherapy prior to surgery without major incident, although it was deeply distressing to see her in so much pain. I felt so useless. *I'm a doctor and I still can't do anything to help her.* All I could do was be there for her emotionally and practically, help her decode medical jargon and advocate for her wherever needed. Bella attended every one of Mum's appointments, supporting her through her cancer journey every step of the way. After the complications from Mum's first chemotherapy treatment, and to ease my mind about her being alone, I helped Mum train Bella to retrieve the mobile phone in case of an emergency. She was getting exceptionally good at this new complex task, making me feel a bit more at ease.

The renovation of the house continued. Managing all the workers' comings and goings, Benni's ongoing health concerns and now Mum's cancer was becoming a real challenge. The business had a few private training clients, so I had income, but being available for Mum was a greater priority. All the minor problems and delays associated with renovating a house just seemed so trivial in the grand scheme of things. However, if I ever wanted to have a functional house, I would have to keep going and make sure it was finished! I wasn't the best version of myself with the builders. With everything going on, delay after delay and soaring cost estimates, it was all pushing my ability to cope to its absolute limits.

In the first week of August 2022, Mum finally had her operation. They called during the operation to advise the cancer had spread to the outside surface of the bowel, so they needed to cut this section of the bowel out and this may lead to a stoma (a poo bag, as Mum affectionately called it). Mum and I spoke openly about her cancer so we had discussed this potential eventuality. Mum expressed she wanted to live, and if that required a "poo bag" she would accept it. I relayed Mum's wishes to the operating team and they cut out the affected part of the bowel and joined up the ends. Thankfully, she didn't end up needing a stoma. I was surprised at how useful it made me feel being able to understand and decode the medical information related to Mum's treatment. For so long it felt like I had to throw away 20 years of work and life experience when I could no longer work in medicine, but I was learning my medical knowledge would become very useful. The transferrable skills from my various roles were also assisting with my work.

This was such a difficult time, and Mum felt so far away in Brisbane. I was looking after Bella so I couldn't just drop in and see how she was going. It must have been such a lonely time for her too, admitted to a huge hospital, having a massive operation and having no family nearby to visit. I was conscious of how challenging this would be for her so a few days post-op, when I knew she would be up to a visit, I took Bella to visit her. I had previously witnessed the healing effects of the dogs on Mum and hoped this would help her focus on recovery so she could get home to Bella.

It was such a relief to see her sitting up and well, and she was so happy to see us. Bella was amazing, putting a smile on the faces of everyone we came across but most of all she made Mum feel better. On August 18, 2022, Mum was discharged. I took her and Bella home to stay with Benni and me for her post-op recovery. She was still having trouble standing up straight because of the massive abdominal wound so she was sent home with a wheelie walker. Within a week of being home, Benni started to pester her, wanting to touch her belly wound.

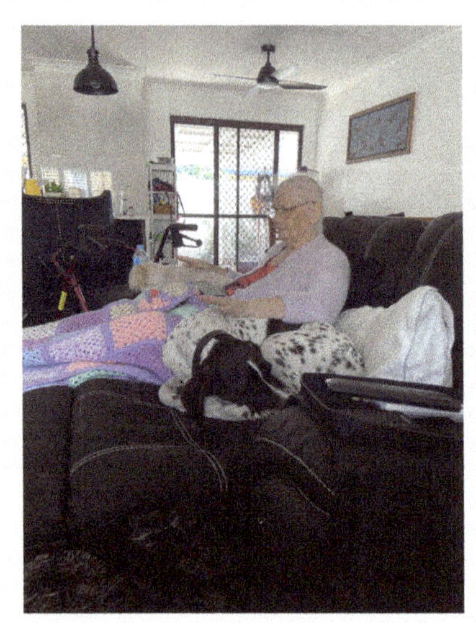

Mum, her wheelie walker and two furry carers

Mum ended up having to put a pillow in front of her wound to discourage Benni from going near it. Once the pillow was in the way, Benni would still nudge it out of the way, leaning heavily on Mum's leg. This is one of Benni's alerting behaviours.

Eventually I said to Mum, "I think Benni is alerting but I'm not sure what to."

Assistance dogs are trained to alert their handlers to specific things like low blood sugar levels or imminent seizures, but Benni had never been trained to alert for wound issues.

After Benni annoyed Mum for the umpteenth time, I asked, "Mum, do you mind if I take a look at the wound?"

"No, why?"

"Maybe Benni's trying to tell us something."

After taking down the dressing, I could see some discoloured fluid coming from the wound site.

"It looks a bit red and it's oozing a bit. Mum, I think you might have an infection." The discharge from the wound was also a bit smelly and offensive. "Maybe that's what Benni's trying to tell us."

We decided to call the GP the next day to arrange a wound check but I checked her temperature as a precaution and she had a fever. With her history of ongoing low immunity, she was advised to call an ambulance if she got a fever post-op. When the ambulance came to take Mum and her raging wound infection away, you could see Benni just looking at us as if to say, "I tried to tell you, but you didn't listen!"

Mum and I were still having a laugh with the paramedics as we relayed the story about not listening to Benni as Mum was being loaded into the ambulance. Two assistance dogs in the family, two experienced handlers/ trainers, and no-one listened to the dog! Once she was on oral antibiotics, she was able to come back home. Mum became quite attached to her wheelie walker over the next week. I eventually had to tell her she wasn't allowed to extend the rental anymore. She was becoming dependant on it but she could walk just fine without it. This became a hilarious recurrent discussion about getting her another wheelie walker well after she had recovered from surgery and was walking several kilometres a day.

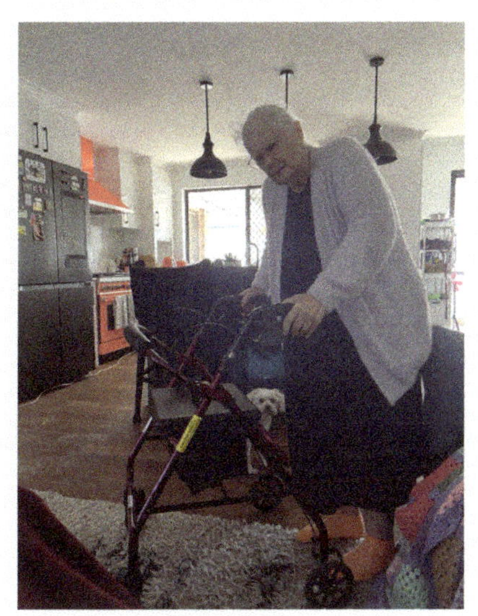

"See? I really need my walker" Hamming it up for the camera

"I'll get my wheelie walker one day – you watch," she said.

After the operation, the wound infection and Mum's recovery period in my home, she went back to her home, wheelie walker free, and settled into the next round of post-op chemotherapy. The histopathology (microscopic results) came back and confirmed Mum had stage 3C (advanced) ovarian cancer.

By September the renovations were taking shape but progress remained slow. My son and his wife were due to come back from overseas and they were supposed to have a unit out the front to stay in but nothing was finished. I felt mounting pressure to try and get this space completed before they arrived. I wanted to provide a comfortable, separate area for them to stay so they would be happy

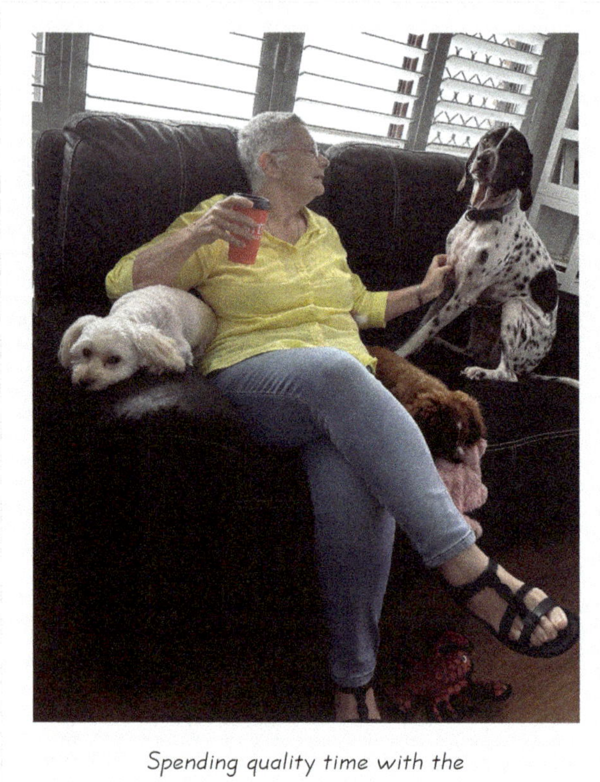

Spending quality time with the dogs she loved so much

and maybe even choose to live nearby. Mum was also selling her little car to upgrade, so I took the opportunity both to help her and to secure a car as a surprise for Eliot, hoping it would give them the independence they needed to make the transition easier. They would arrive by the end of October so the pressure to get the front finished was accumulating, but the work simply wasn't completed in time. It had been a long and stressful year, so I was really looking forward to seeing them.

I felt a lot of self-imposed pressure to make everything just right for my son and of course nothing went to plan! The unit out the front wasn't anywhere near ready, my house was still a construction zone, which came with all the inconveniences of a building site, and our whole household was struck down with Covid, making all three of us very sick. Mum was finally having a treatment break and thankfully didn't contract Covid. I asked the builders to put in a dishwasher instead of an additional cupboard to make things more comfortable in the unit but it would never get used. Amid the building disruptions, illness and general exhaustion – and with Benni frustrating everyone with her medication-induced food obsession – my best laid plans unravelled. Eliot moved to a new home base hundreds of kilometres away and Mum went away to spend time with her sister, Aunty K, for Christmas. I was alone and feeling like my world was falling apart again. They say the things you fear most you focus on and this makes them more likely to happen. My greatest fear was ending up completely alone. My mind spiralled, convincing me that my worst fears had finally come true. *Now I'm truly alone. Everyone I ever cared about is gone.* Of course, this wasn't the case; since 2014 it's just where my brain goes when these things happen.

That Christmas was the loneliest time in my entire life. I did a lot of soul searching. As a precaution I again engaged with the GP and the psychologist. I was quite baffled by my response to this situation as I was generally very happy and worked hard to be quite regulated in my responses to things. My impatience and uncharacteristic anger during the renovations were signs I wasn't coping under the pressure. I started to understand my brain was again overwhelmed by circumstance and had developed a default system. Whenever I experienced what I perceived as a loss, I would struggle to cope with it. It was almost automatic, like it was built in, and each time I would have to reason with it and talk myself through it. This took me by surprise. *How did I end up here, so completely and utterly alone? Did I actually die in 2014? Is this some cruel alternative reality? When is this misery ever going to stop? Why am I thinking this way? I have so much to live for!*

Once again, through my tears, Benni was there, reliably providing comfort. She again gave me reasons to get out of bed in the morning. It was up to me to get myself through this period. *You have to stop*

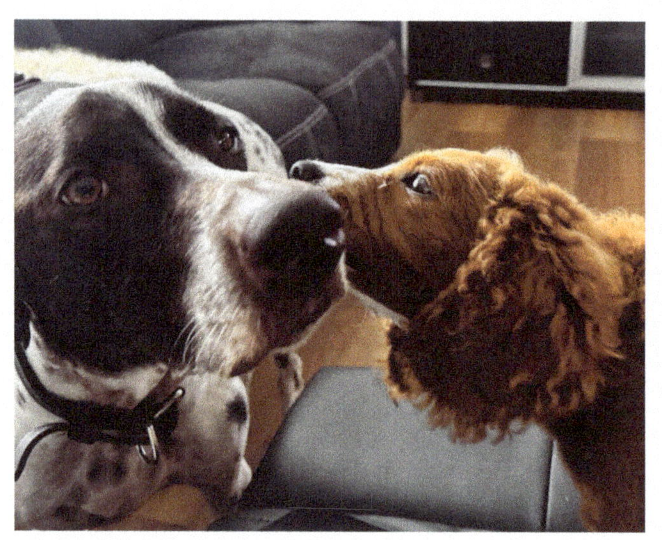

Freya bringing joy back to Benni's life

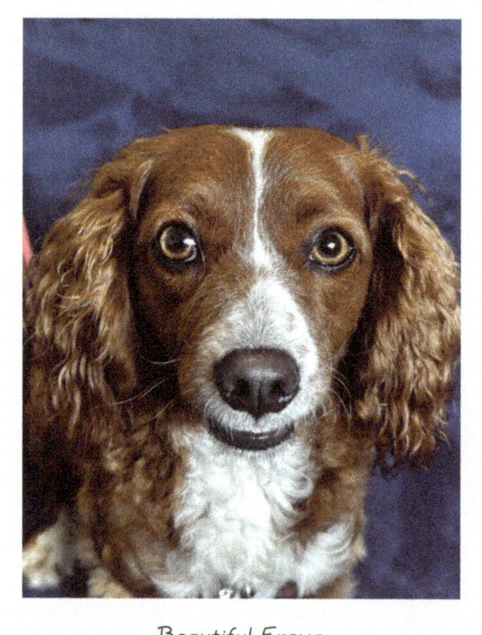

Beautiful Freya

thinking every time you have an unpleasant experience or loss that you're faulty in some way. You'll get through this. As a child, it always felt to me like I was the family scapegoat and, as such, I was conditioned from childhood to believe there was something fundamentally wrong with me. If there was a disagreement, it always seemed to be my fault in some way. If someone was unhappy with me, it always felt like a direct risk to my safety. PTSD also makes you feel like everything's a threat to your safety even when it clearly isn't.

I needed to approach this period of my life differently. I worked so hard to recover from PTSD, to change any dysfunctional coping styles, but, clearly, I needed to work harder. I started to investigate courses again. So many things were out of my control in this time, so I needed to focus on what I could control. I found a 12-month course in animal-assisted psychotherapy and enrolled. I looked into a counselling diploma and enrolled. I tried to find an assistance dog training course but there wasn't one. It was time to start a new phase of life, accepting my choices were contributing to my difficulties. I needed to focus again on making better choices, becoming a better version of myself.

I wanted to help other people with similar struggles in life. I also needed to consider Benni's needs. She had an awful few years with seizures and medications. Her illness meant she was no longer able to work as an assistance dog, so she was really bored. Benni also seemed to be a little down. She stopped doing zoomies and life with her seizure disorder was very difficult at times. I got Benni a friend, a Cavoodle called Freya, who was full of life with a lot of love to give. Freya brought some joy back into Benni's life and she even started to do zoomies again. I closed ranks and started to focus on the dogs and this new stage of life, with the start dates for both courses looming. It was time to simply accept where things were in my life and let go of the things I couldn't control. This was the start of personal integration and prioritising peace.

PEACE

To experience peace in my life every day I'm alive
Now that would be a worthy goal towards which I could strive
It has been an elusive endeavour, unattainable thus far
Perhaps I've been wishing on exactly the wrong star
Striving towards my goals, I had always worked so hard
Only to find I had been dealt every single wrong card
I tried to find it in my job and in so many other things
But peace is actually not what all that stuff brings
Peace is not a destination, not a place to arrive
It's that feeling of warmth you get deep inside
When your values are on display, you're feeling whole
Peace will arrive from deep within your soul
You won't have to find it, it will be wherever you reside
Protecting it is one rule by which you'll have to abide
You see, peace is a rare commodity, everyone else wants it too
But if you give all your peace to others, there will be none left for you

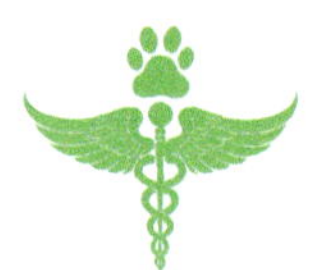

The animal-assisted psychotherapy (AAP) course was a 12-month weekly Zoom commitment with significant assessment requirements at the end of the course. It was offered by an organisation called the Equine & Animal Assisted Psychotherapy Institute. I enrolled in this course so I could effectively help others experience the same transformative relationships with dogs I had. I hoped the combination of the counselling course and the AAP course would allow me to achieve what my young clients had inspired me to do, combine my love of dog training with therapy. I had no idea these courses would also be transformative for me.

The AAP course was based on a form of therapy I was unfamiliar with called Gestalt therapy. This was a humanistic, person-centred kind of approach to therapy that involved developing self-awareness, taking personal responsibility and integrating the 'disowned' parts of self.[4] This was such a new concept for me and I soaked it up like a sponge. I wasn't just learning it; I was applying it to myself. Each week we also included our animal and applied this approach to the interactions we had with them too. Benni was loving her new life with Freya and enjoying participating in these sessions. This was very much in line with my personal values, so I really enjoyed the content. Mum was in remission so things settled for a while, giving me a chance to relax a little and enjoy what I was learning. I was still training assistance dogs and trying to find the right course to legitimise my work. The counselling course was running alongside the AAP course and it was just as interesting. I was taking a deep dive back into the theories that underpin our understanding of human and

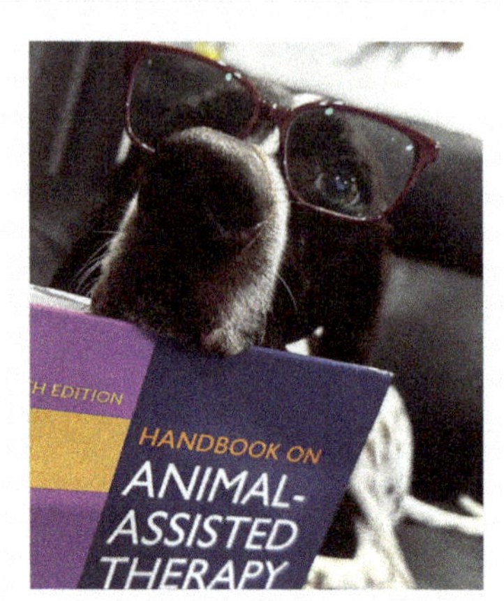

We literally studied together!

coincidentally dog behaviour, with many studies involved in these theories being performed on dogs.

Somewhere in the middle of these courses, I realised something: my brain was working again. Assessments weren't too much of a challenge and my frustration tolerance was building. My brain was starting to heal from the years of trauma it had suffered. It was a surprise then when I started to get physically ill. I had previously contracted Covid and months later it was still messing with my system. I was having palpitations, my heart was racing if I stood for long periods, I was extremely physically fatigued and one night I woke up with half my vision missing on my right side. This resolved, leaving behind a headache that lasted days. I thought I had Long Covid Syndrome, but it was time to see the doctor to find out what was wrong with me.

As a retired doctor and someone with a mental health history, I absolutely hate going to the doctor but this time I felt it was a necessary evil. Luckily, I had a great GP that helped me go down several rabbit holes to find out what was going on. The GP found my blood pressure was elevated at night when it should be low and started me on some medication to control it. There were a few little lesions in my brain that were consistent with normal age-related changes and there was nothing else to find but I just kept getting sicker. I told her it felt a lot like serotonin syndrome. I would get an overwhelming sensation of dread followed by flushing, with my face going red, I would have trouble breathing, sometimes I was itchy all over, and this could be followed by any number of other weird symptoms. I was regularly experiencing an all-over body itch, numbness and a burning sensation in my feet and hands, difficulty breathing, a lump in my throat, diarrhoea and a fast heart rate.

I began to keep a symptom diary so I could track what was happening for myself. I knew from past experience that having a mental health diagnosis and weird symptoms often seemed to increase the risk of being dismissed, but I knew there was something physically wrong with me. I'd experienced what I perceived to be medical gaslighting before (where the doctor decides your subjective experience and symptoms aren't real) and I really didn't want to experience the deep sense of helplessness that comes with it again. I developed a few allergies after the liver injury in 2014 and some of the symptoms were consistent with allergy. Since 2014 I have developed so many allergies I lost count, so I had a lot of experience with allergic reactions – from mild hives all the way up to life-threatening anaphylaxis.

I experienced another couple of weird episodes of visual loss and, after seeing an ophthalmologist (eye doctor), they were diagnosed as atypical migraines. I felt like these things were all linked so I spent some more time looking into them myself. I put on my doctor cap and dived deep into the literature, trying to find out what was wrong with me. I developed symptoms consistent with peripheral nerve damage and had seen a neurologist. Tests still didn't show what was going on. After a couple of episodes of dangerously high blood pressure, I ended up in hospital being investigated for a potential occult (hidden) cancer. I knew from my medical training that a paraneoplastic syndrome (a weird cluster of symptoms caused by the release of hormones or other substances from a tumour somewhere) was a possibility and wanted to have this excluded. I was still studying and trying to keep up with my courses but started to fall behind. They told me they thought this may be a paraneoplastic syndrome and I may have a very small cancer in my intestines, causing a condition called carcinoid syndrome.

Now this is a very rare condition, and this wasn't the first time I was told I may have a carcinoid tumour. It had been a consideration around the time I'd had several episodes of serotonin syndrome. I began to fear I may actually have cancer. I talked to Mum and reluctantly decided to tell Eliot what was going on in case it did turn out to be cancer. Eliot came up to visit, which was lovely. With Mum's diagnosis and my anxiety flaring, I was really frightened and spending time with Eliot was healing. I was still doing my own research since the one thing that seemed to be working well was my brain. I was discharged for more investigations with the suggestion this may be a small intestinal cancer.

But something told me it wasn't cancer. In my extensive research into the combination of symptoms, I came across a condition called Mast Cell Activation Syndrome, or MCAS for short. It explained all my symptoms and a decade of my life finally made sense. In MCAS you're oversensitive to histamine, your immune system overreacts to medications and other triggers, and the response can vary depending on your circulating histamine levels.[5]

Histamine is a chemical found in many foods and is stored and released by immune cells called mast cells in allergic reactions. It's hard to get a formal diagnosis with MCAS because you need to have your histamine levels checked while you are experiencing anaphylaxis. Diagnosis is often made based on clinical symptoms. Because it's such an unusual condition, I felt my symptoms might not be well understood within standard care pathways, so I sought out a functional medicine GP with experience in MCAS.

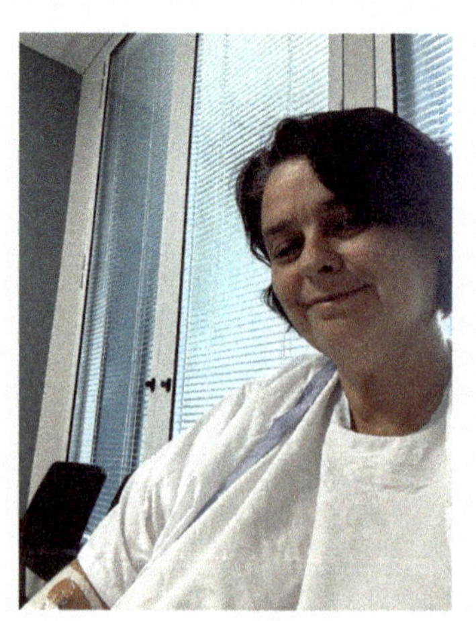

Feeling ordinary and red-faced in an MCAS flare

After an almost two-hour consult, reviewing all the recent investigation results, collecting a lot more bloods and completing a directed questionnaire, it became clear that MCAS was the most likely explanation for my symptoms. I was informed that my recurrent presentations were likely atypical episodes of anaphylaxis. I went on a low histamine diet, some supplements, some strong antihistamines, and ceased the blood pressure medication, which coincided with resolution of the neuropathy symptoms (peripheral neuropathy is a recognised side effect of some blood pressure medications). I started to feel a lot better. We discussed how important it was to regulate my immune system not only with diet and medication but also through emotional regulation. Stress is a major trigger for MCAS and I needed to learn how to manage it better. My peace had to take priority, as my health now depended on it.

After getting a few extensions on my work I was finally able to catch up again. The content was fascinating. I was now really invested in doing the work not only so I could help others but also so I could help my immune system become more regulated. One of the wonderful parts of Gestalt therapy is the integration or acceptance of the parts of yourself that you have previously rejected.[6] My understanding of this is we're often told or decide there's something wrong with us or our coping styles, then go to therapy to fix it. This AAP course was telling me something different; to acknowledge those things about ourselves and accept how, at some point in our lives, they served a purpose. They were how we survived whatever situation we were in.[7] This was a complete transformation of how I saw my last 10 years, including the mistakes and fractures in relationships.

Whatever coping mechanism I used to get through the difficult things in my life, no matter how dysfunctional it was perceived to be, it got me through. I was still here! It had served an important function at the time but didn't necessarily serve me well now. We also learnt about mindfulness and awareness in self and of others in the course. Mindfulness training was not new to me, but I spent time deepening my understanding, learning to spend quiet time just feeling the sensations my body was offering me and honouring them as forms of communication to my brain.

We learnt about the cycles of experience and how our styles of interacting with others can interrupt your experience of the world, preventing you from feeling joy, sorrow or other authentic emotions.[8] Authenticity was also discussed, and I realised I had spent so much of my life trying to be the version of me that kept the people around me happy (and therefore me safe). In the process, I neglected some of the authentic parts of myself and my personal experience of life was suffering as a result. I was brought back to the idea that I can only control how *I* think, feel and act and I cannot control what others think of me, how they feel or how they act. My focus shifted to what was in my control and I was genuinely able to let go of what was out of my control. I started to focus on my values of trust, unconditional love, ethics, compassion, security, honesty and commitment in relationships.

Commitment in relationships was interesting as I found a dichotomy here within myself. I was committed to my relationships and would have stayed committed for life but my need for compassion and care at a time of extreme vulnerability, and therefore this value, was more important to me. I learnt there are times in life when your values will conflict with one another and you must choose between them. These are the times that tell you what you need to know about yourself. I valued compassion over commitment, and I was okay with this discovery. I decided my first priority, and number one value, was going to be peace. I believe with peace comes compassion for others. My new internal mantra would become *My peace comes first*. I developed a deep desire to help others with similar experiences and share what helped me get through times of extreme difficulty. Only from a place of peace and healing can you truly be of service to others.

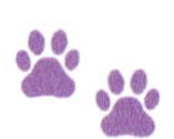

Benni's epilepsy stabilised for a while, but her health took a dive while I was doing my final assessment for the diploma of counselling. Without warning, Benni had a massive seizure on the evening of July 3, 2023. I called Mum to come and look after Freya as she was still a young puppy at the time. Benni suffered another seizure while Mum was on her way. I called the vet who advised to bring her in if she had a third seizure, so I got everything ready to leave. She had another seizure just as Mum arrived. I gave her a dose of the emergency medication (midazolam) up her nose before I carried her out the door. The vet was a 25-minute drive away and I was very nervous getting in the car. I secured her in her seatbelt and made sure the child lock was on the door in case another seizure came on while I was driving.

I drew up another dose of her emergency medication and kept it by my side. Sure enough, Benni had another seizure about halfway to the vet. I quickly stopped to give her a second dose of this emergency medication then drove as fast and as safely as I could to the vet. I used the voice-activated call feature on my car to call on the way to let them know how serious it was. As we arrived and I handed her over to the nurse, she was seizing again without recovering in between. The vet explained, and I knew from my medical training, this was status epilepticus (prolonged or recurrent seizure activity that won't stop) and if they couldn't stop the seizures she could die. As expected, I was faced with a form and a massive deposit. This time I was prepared with the Benni Fund and there was more than $5,000 in it. So I told them to do whatever it took to save her. Benni had been my purpose for so long, I wanted and needed her to be okay.

I could hear every tick of the clock as I waited for what seemed like an eternity before they came out to see me.

"You can come in and see her now if you like."

They talked to me about how serious status epilepticus is because her brain was deprived of oxygen for a long time.

"We won't be able to tell just yet but she could have sustained some brain damage. We have started her on a drug to reduce her brain swelling." They gently raised the possibility of putting her to sleep. "It might be time to consider quality of life and what's in her best interests."

I knelt on the floor next to the crate she was in. The hum of all the machines keeping her alive was deafening, with infusions to reduce her brain swelling, to stop her seizures and to correct some nasty imbalances in her blood all running through drips in her front legs. She looked up at me with her droopy but understanding eyes. She knew we were all just trying to help her but she also knew she was desperately unwell.

I looked deeply into her sedated little eyes, put my hand on her paw and gently said, "Mummy's got you. I'm not ready. Benni, you have to fight." I turned to the vet and told him I wanted all treatment possible and if she had brain damage, we would deal with that after.

"Okay then." He looked surprised but gave an understanding nod as I turned around to go back to the front desk.

I loved this dog more than I could describe to any human being. We had been through some of the toughest times in life together and we always had each other's backs. I signed another form stating I wanted

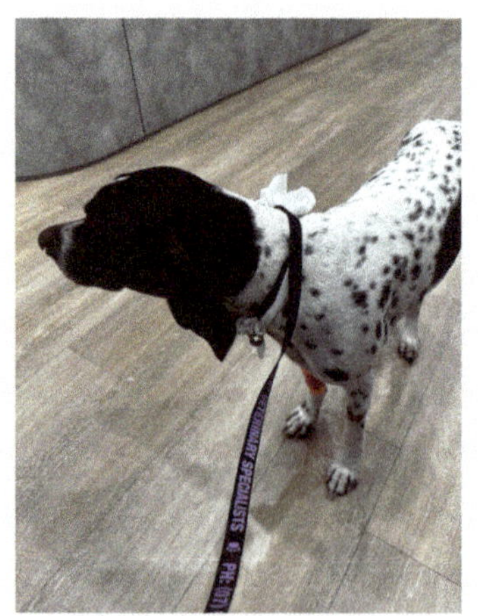

Benni recovering from status with a seizure bell around her neck

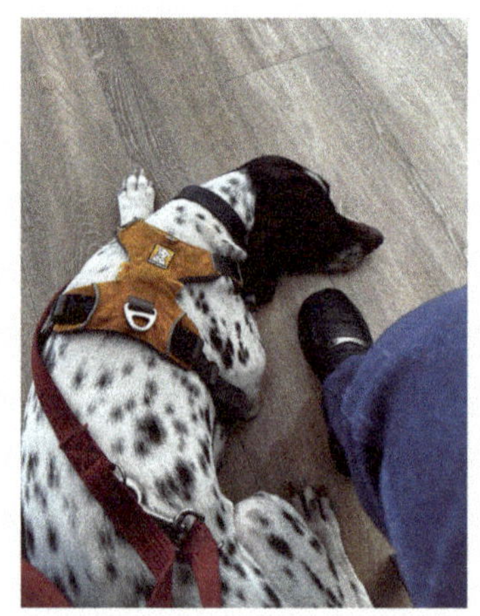

The day I got to take her home

full resuscitation if she deteriorated and confirming I understood this could be very expensive. I paid my huge deposit, went out to the car, slumped into the driver's seat and, sobbing, I begged gods I'm not sure I believed in not to take her away!

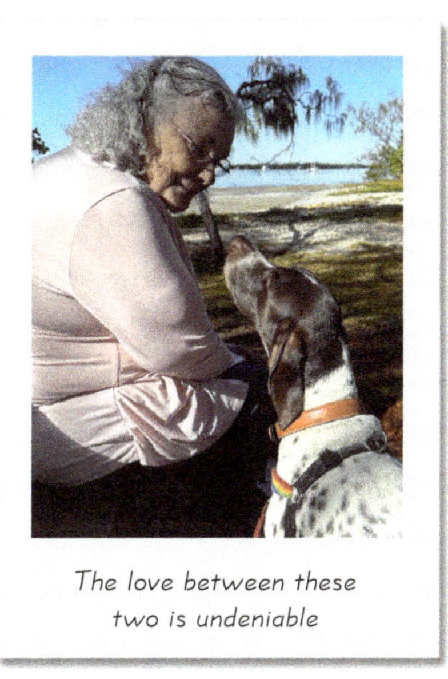

The love between these two is undeniable

The specialist vet took such great care of my special little Benni. After two days of admission she was finally able to come home. They were able to stabilise her but she was prescribed yet another new medication. She was now taking 10 tablets a day for her epilepsy. This medication also required a loading dose (higher initial dose). As a result, for a while she was very wobbly on her feet, unable to get up, mobilise or go to the toilet without help, and she wet herself a few times. Mum returned from a trip away and developed Covid so she couldn't help me care for Benni as she had always done. However, she was very supportive and empathetic about beautiful Benni, as she loved her almost as much as I did.

Benni recovered fairly quickly from the admission but there was some residual back leg weakness and minor deficits we figured were from the prolonged period her brain endured without oxygen. Within a month or two she was back to her cheeky, food-stealing, undie-tossing self only with wobbly back legs. This new medication proved to be a godsend. Her seizures stopped and she was able to have some quality of life again, running around annoying Freya. When she was fully recovered, she was back at home with me ready to start her new role as a part-time therapy dog. Benni was so intelligent and therefore so bored when she wasn't working. She needed a purpose and working as a part-time therapy dog from my home would mean she could provide valuable support for those in need, retreating to the peace of her backyard whenever she needed to. During her recovery, I had to seriously consider what I would do if faced with the same situation again. I believe Benni will let me know when she's had enough of the suffering. I looked into the necessary services so if anything happened again, I could support her to die peacefully in her own home.

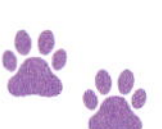

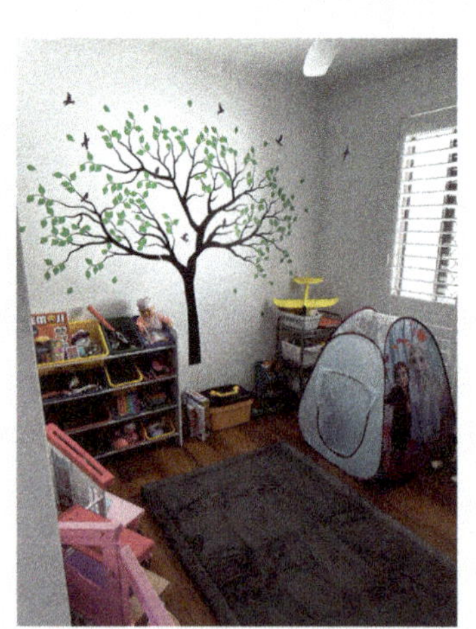

The beautiful P3 Play Paws Psychotherapy playroom

Despite some hiccups along the way, I finally completed the diploma of counselling, the AAP course and, somewhere in between, heard about a treatment modality called Child Centred Play Therapy (CCPT). Since many of the dogs I was training were working with children, I was also deeply interested in CCPT as a therapeutic modality. I completed a course in CCPT as well and opened a new arm of my little business in August 2023 called P3 Play Paws Psychotherapy. The unit I developed out the front of my home became our new home base. Benni, Freya and I, and occasionally Bella, went to work providing trauma-informed, ethical animal-assisted interventions, including CCPT, AAP and counselling. I was still training dogs for people with disabilities and looking for the perfect course to legitimise this practice, but there was still nothing out there. I was coming from a healed place within myself and finally felt able to be of service to others.

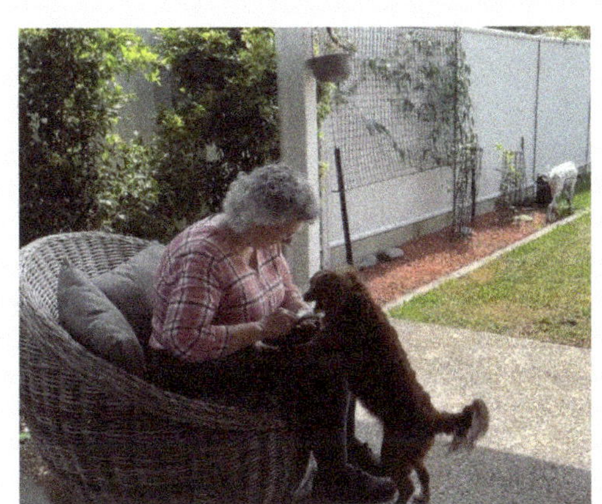

Mum with Freya on the day we filmed my assessment and after being told, "It's back"

Mum agreed to be my volunteer for the final video assessment for the AAP course. However, when she was diagnosed with a recurrence of her cancer, I told her I would get someone else. Mum refused, insisting on continuing with this assessment for me, giving me just a few specific questions to avoid asking. My final assessment in AAP was a 30-minute, video-recorded animal-assisted psychotherapy session with Mum talking about what it felt like to have a recurrence of her cancer while interacting with Benni. The video was so powerful for me. The organisation later sought Mum's approval to use it for teaching purposes, which she happily consented to. This was an incredibly privileged position to be in and it gave me some insight into the internal anguish she had experienced throughout her cancer diagnosis and the devastation of being told, "It's back."

Mum helped me set up for the opening of the new little business and was always there cheering me on no matter what I did in my adult life. Mum would also come and pretend to be a stranger when we were practising polite greetings with assistance dog trainees, so many of my clients got to know and love her. Mum was nervous about this recurrence and the resulting treatment. She had peripheral neuropathy (painful nerve damage) from her previous chemotherapy, which had led to dose reductions in previous treatments. Consequently, the regime was changed to minimise this side effect for her and ensure the treatment was effective. Like many chemotherapeutics, this new drug came with an awful list of unspeakable potential side effects, but it was the next best thing to the one that caused her peripheral neuropathy. She tolerated this drug well but her cell counts were really suffering. The bone marrow makes many of the important cells in your body and chemotherapy often kills bone marrow. Mum had several more episodes of low neutrophils and low platelets (platelets are the little cells responsible for effective clotting), requiring treatment, but otherwise was doing okay.

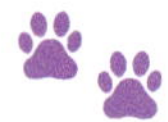

In 2024 life was good, the business was going well, Mum was on an oral maintenance therapy because her platelets kept coming back low, but she was otherwise well. I expressed concern to the oncologist about secondary blood cancer (myelodysplastic disorder or leukaemia) from chemotherapy and she checked for this. All was good so we relaxed again and got on with life.

My little business was thriving, and I was absolutely loving it. I was developing my own treatment modality I now call Canine Integrative

Relational Therapy (CIRT). I kept thinking: *This isn't work. I didn't know you could enjoy work this much.* I was contributing in a meaningful way, making a difference while working with my beautiful dogs in my home, and even on long days I would walk out with a smile. I was coming from a healed place within me, consistent with my core values. *This is what they mean when they say if you love what you do you'll never work a day in your life.*

I was working for myself, which afforded me the flexibility to arrange my schedule around Mum's appointments. For most of her treatments I was also able to drop her off and pick her up. My father had returned from New Zealand and was staying very close by, though I remained completely unaware of his presence. Years earlier I told him I would never pursue him again, and I remained steadfast in that resolve. It seemed symbolic of the distance between us. He was so close, according to him even attending lunches within walking distance from my house, while I remained completely unaware of his presence. I believe this is one of the many features of such a dysfunctional family, something I no longer felt interested in being involved in. There's always someone on the outer in a dysfunctional family and I now felt comfortable being the proverbial "black sheep".

There also seemed to be some sort of drama attached to being around Dad. He was constantly struggling with something and it felt like there was some level of competition for his attention from those around him. My peace was my priority. I wasn't upset, jealous or angry when I found out he had been nearby – just a little surprised. Not at the fact I wasn't invited but at how often so many people just seemed to go along with his behaviours without speaking up. I guess this comes from having to survive that behaviour yourself. When you're dealing with someone as volatile and divisive as my father was, you need to self-preserve. This was something I often struggled with, both in my relationship with Dad and my work in medicine. I've never been able to stand by and watch someone be mistreated or excluded without speaking up. In the past, this tendency often came with consequences, but it's part of myself I have since come to embrace and even value.

I guess it's understandable no-one around him seemed able to speak up about exclusion of a family member from these gatherings. Over time, I also recognised people like my father were very charismatic and convincing, so they were always surrounded by people who seemed to readily agree with them. Those affected frequently seem isolated (deliberately or otherwise) from anyone who might offer a different perspective. I now not only understand this dynamic but have come to a place of radical acceptance, seeing these patterns as part of the self that was serving Dad and the people around him at the time, keeping them safe and connected. I didn't need to feel isolated or alone anymore. My peace was more valuable than any interaction with him or inclusion in any gatherings would ever be. I learned to enjoy his company, when it was available, choosing to release any lingering anger or resentment. I've come to believe we are all equal, just people doing the best we can with the tools we have available to us at the time.

As always, I was still on the lookout for a magic course to help me on my mission to become an accredited assistance dog training organisation, and it finally became available in 2024. I enrolled in the Certificate IV in Animal Behaviour and Assistance Dog Training, offered by Hanrob College, and started working away at the requirements. This would require many hours of placement and many written assessments. I was finally ready for this challenge, determined to finish within six months instead of 12. Knowing how unpredictable Mum's condition could be, things could change at any time. I wanted to be ready for any potential eventuality.

It was difficult to secure placement, but I finally found an amazing charity called In The Paws of Angels. The beautiful founder, Samantha Gallagher, trainer John and volunteer Di took me under their wings. I felt so fortunate to have found these wonderful people. Sam, John, Di and all the volunteers have become firm friends. It's funny how you attract such beautiful, genuine people when you're living to your values. I was loving this course, loving spending time with these beautiful people, and I was breezing through it. I also started to look into spirituality again as it felt like I had come full circle, back to the early days where spirituality was part of my everyday life.

This time it was different. I fundamentally no longer bought into the model that we're all flawed and need fixing. In my clinical practice I made sure my clients and their families also understood I didn't believe in the "broken" model. I believe we are all imperfectly perfect and can work with our strengths to improve our personal circumstances. I now believed all the parts of me, including the ones I didn't necessarily like, were important and needed to be integrated instead of removed to be authentic. I also came to understand how integral my relationships with dogs (and other animals) were in my life. These beautiful creatures were so much more than pets. They can think and reason for themselves, and have an incredible, innate ability to offer unconditional love, compassion and support.

GRIEF

I thought I knew grief, but the truth makes me cross
There's so many different ways to experience loss
Loss of a marriage, loss of a hard-fought career
Loss of a relationship with a child you hold so dear
Loss of financial security, loss of meaning in life
Loss of your role as a partner, husband or wife
Each time there's a loss, the heart breaks just a little
The shaking ground below you starts to feel so brittle
Then comes the death of a loved one or maybe even two
In the mirror you see an unfamiliar face staring back at you
What happened to that confident doctor, wife, mother and child
There's nothing left of who I was, my sense of self exiled
Reinvention would be the only potential for cure
Giving up, a constant option with significant allure
But just as the sun rises and sets at the end of each day
Life must go on, somehow, I just have to find a way
With all the strength I can muster from deep within my soul
I need to work on the few things that are left in my control
So, with whatever there is left of what used to be me
I will try to keep moving forward, persistence the key
One day, I'm told, the pain will gradually subside
But with each episode of grief I die a little, on the inside

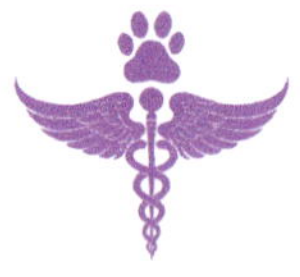

The course was going well, and Mum was still on her oral maintenance hormone-based treatment. The scans still showed some persistent but stable disease and her platelets were still too low to have any more chemotherapy at this point. However, the caravan park she was living in was closing down, and they let her know she'd have to move on. This was a blow for Mum – the last thing she needed was housing insecurity. I reassured her she would have a home with me and I would move the business out to a commercial lease if necessary. One random day in June, I received a call to advise me Dad was in hospital after a fainting episode. Dad had significant and widespread cardiovascular disease with multiple prior serious complications. In medicine we refer to people like Dad as "vasculopaths" – people with significant vascular (blood vessel) pathology who are high risk for recurrent vascular complications.

I was surprised to find they were treating him for simple dehydration. Dad was complaining of abdominal pain, worried about his graft (mesh repair) from a previous dissecting abdominal aortic aneurysm (a blowout of a major abdominal blood vessel wall that was leaking blood). Just one of the many serious cardiovascular complications Dad had suffered. He asked the medical team to organise a scan to check this graft and I reiterated this to the staff. I made sure the junior doctor was aware of Dad's complicated medical history and need to be reviewed by a senior clinician. He was assessed by the senior clinician as planned and discharged. Dad was given a referral for an abdominal CT (Computed Tomography) scan so he could have this done outside the hospital. Things settled so I heard no more about Dad's pain and I thought no more of his health at this time. It always seemed unusual for

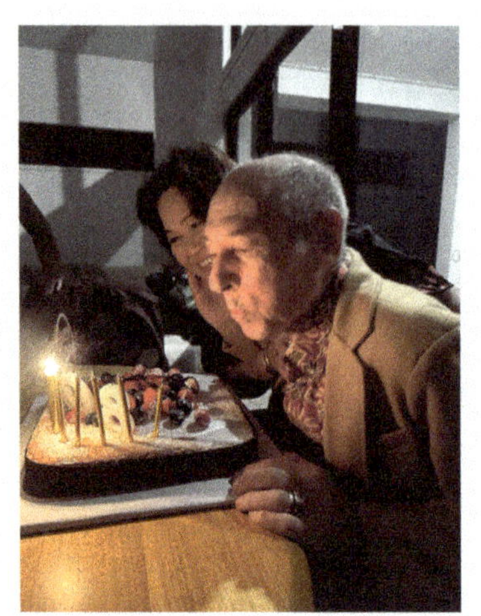

Dad at his 80th birthday party

me to be invited to family events, so I was quite surprised to get an invite to Dad's 80th birthday party and agreed to attend.

The party was lovely, and you could tell by his demeanour he was really enjoying it too. However, there seemed to be an air of finality in his speech. I sensed he was feeling his age and potentially his mortality.

Dad and Nang were now trying to get their house (a big yacht) back from New Zealand. In September they made a valiant attempt with some very capable crew taking on the challenge. As with many things with Dad, this led to a significant incident, ending in a broken rudder, a boat that was useless out at sea, one crew member being rescued from the vessel, and the remaining crew having to limp it back to New Zealand with the Coast Guard monitoring the situation. According to Dad, if the crew had to abandon the vessel, under maritime law it could be salvaged by someone else, giving them costly salvage rights over the vessel. It was a very stressful time for all concerned. This wasn't just their only asset – this was their home. Now, thanks to the amazing crew's efforts, it was broken but safely back in port. However, it was still thousands of kilometres away.

The stress was taking its toll on Dad's health. On Friday October 11, I was back in hospital visiting him after he collapsed at home going to the bathroom. There was some debate about whether this was another vascular event, but scans revealed a large mass partially blocking his large bowel along with some other concerning findings. The doctors advised us he had a bowel obstruction (blockage) likely secondary to bowel cancer. If it was bowel cancer, it looked like it had already spread through the abdomen, potentially into his lungs. I knew how serious this was. He was unlikely to be around for much longer.

It was a shock to me how advanced the cancer was already. I patiently waited to hear any more news. On Monday, October 14 he was discharged, with the obstruction thought to be resolved. As a preventative measure, and to ensure I maintained my peace, I contacted my psychologist and GP to ensure I would have support around issues relating to Dad's illness. Given the complex nature of my relationship with Dad, this time I wanted to be proactive and manage any distress ahead of time rather than waiting for a crisis to occur.

Dad was scheduled to return for a scope (a camera that is put into the bowel) and biopsy to confirm the diagnosis. By Saturday, October 19, all the familiar signs of a bowel obstruction had returned. He was back in hospital, though this time quite unstable. The medical team decided they would have to operate to prevent a bowel perforation (rupture) as the obstruction had caused dangerous dilation of other parts of the bowel. I waited in a tiny corner of the hospital with Nang while he was having his operation. They advised he may end up with a stoma. The lovely doctor was aware of my medical training and gave me the professional courtesy of agreeing to call with an update after the operation. I felt the weight of responsibility around communication of medical information to family, the gravity of the situation and the risks being very clear in my mind but probably not as well understood by the people around me. In my view, this was a disastrous diagnosis. I sensed it would be a rough ride ahead. It felt like emotions were running high in those around me, yet I was able to maintain a sense of calm. I attribute this to the peace I cultivated over the past year and the ongoing practice of emotional regulation.

After several tense hours of waiting, the doctor finally called. It was official. There was extensive, metastatic (spread) bowel cancer, and although Dad had undergone a bowel resection (removal of the diseased bowel), they were able to join it back up again so he didn't need a stoma. I was quite surprised, but felt this was a good outcome for such a horrible diagnosis. He would spend a day or so in ICU and then be transferred back to the ward.

It wasn't long before he deteriorated again.

After Dad came back to the ward, he gradually began to decline. At one point I believed he may have another obstruction or, worse, a leak from where they joined up the two ends of the bowel. Dad was progressively getting worse. When he developed a fever and the scan confirmed he had a leak at the join, it became apparent to me he would have to go back to theatre and have a stoma. I chose to stay again to await the outcome of the surgery, though this time he was going to be much weaker and, in my opinion, likely septic from the leak. The doctor again agreed to call and inform me of the outcome after the operation. I felt genuinely grateful for this professional courtesy, as I personally don't believe it was part of their usual practice. The wait felt incredibly long, but finally the phone rang. Nang was right next to me, overhearing the beginning of the conversation. I moved away so I could hear more clearly as Nang was crying. From what the doctor told me, Dad suffered a cardiac event (heart attack) during the procedure and things were touch and go (the part Nang overheard) for a while. In my understanding, he had become so unstable they couldn't close his wound, so he would need another operation to facilitate this when he was more stable. Dad was admitted to ICU, and sedated with machines supporting his breathing. I was told we could briefly go and see him if we wanted to.

When I walked in with Nang they informed us he had sepsis, was recovering from a heart attack, and was on special medications to bring up his blood pressure and manage his cardiac issues. It felt as though there were tubes everywhere – a breathing tube, multiple lines, machines managing nearly all his functions and what I understood to be an open wound covered by a blue piece of sponge. I had experience with critically ill patients and felt the ICU was the best place for someone this sick, but I knew this was new for other family members. Understandably, Nang was inconsolable at the very sight of Dad this unwell. I had a quick cry myself before returning to what I saw as my role – a medically trained daughter trying to stay grounded.

A few years earlier, with all the complex family dynamics, I doubt I could have regulated myself this well. I found myself in an intensely emotional environment, surrounded by deeply distressed people, while trying to process the fact that this was my dad. I was acutely aware of how serious his condition seemed to be and, to me, it was a very real possibility he may not survive the recovery period. At the same time, I had great confidence in the ICU staff and their ability to keep him alive for now. I felt it was essential for me to stay calm and regulated so I could remain an informed, steady, practical support for those around me. I was also aware of the importance of looking after my own wellbeing, which for me meant actively managing my autonomic nervous system (fight or flight), which could easily take over in such a stressful situation.

Dad remained sedated and intubated in ICU until his sepsis settled and his heart and blood pressure were stable enough to tolerate closing the wound. I visited regularly to keep updated about his condition. He went back for his third and final surgery. I was a bit more hopeful he would survive this and end up back on the ward and perhaps even get to go home. After the closure the histopathology came back and the doctors advised Dad of the results. I was visiting with Nang and, with both the doctor's and Dad's permission, I asked for a copy. Even though it was full of medical jargon, reading between the lines, I felt I could piece together the terrible story it told. The report stated that Dad's cancer was very aggressive, having invaded local blood vessels and nerves, and from what I could tell all the distant samples had also come back positive. His prognosis looked very poor. I felt he wasn't going to be alive for much longer and, at this point, it seemed like I was the only person who fully grasped this reality. Carrying this belief and knowing I would eventually have to share it was a heavy burden. The hospital staff seemed to be dancing around the elephant in the room with soft wording, and I imagine this was their way of giving everyone time to come to terms with the dramatic events of the past couple of weeks.

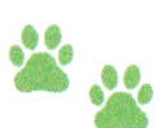

On one of my many visits to Dad in the ICU, Nang had to leave. I was waiting to get a medical update so she wanted me to stay with Dad. Once Nang left, Dad reached out, held my hand and proceeded to give me the greatest gift I ever received from him – his approval. He pulled my hand towards him as if to say come closer, squeezing it tight as I leaned in. He made direct eye contact with me and, holding my gaze, said,

"I'm so proud to call you a Ware."

This was his family name and my maiden name.

"Proud to be one, Dad."

The interaction brought a nearby nurse to tears and I thought: *If only she knew.* I'd fought for so long in my younger life to get his approval and never received it. In this moment he didn't have to give me this. It was a conscious choice and he waited until we were alone, so it was just for me! This is a moment in time that closed so many previous chapters of my life and created an incredible sense of clarity for me. While I didn't need his approval anymore, I was still able to understand, have compassion for him and fully appreciate the gravity of this moment.

As soon as Dad was able, he asked me what the histopathology really said, asking me to be completely honest. Using more frank language, I relayed what the doctors had said, "You have advanced bowel cancer, Dad. It's already spread to your lungs and all through your abdomen. They took out what they could but there's still cancer left behind. They couldn't get it all. The cancer you have is quite aggressive and nasty, and the prognosis isn't good."

He took it all in and then said, "I'm going to beat this – you watch." He was so determined and I didn't want to say any more or oppose his desire to fight. *Dad's very strong, they have new drugs for treatment all the time, so we'll just wait and see what the oncology team have to say.*

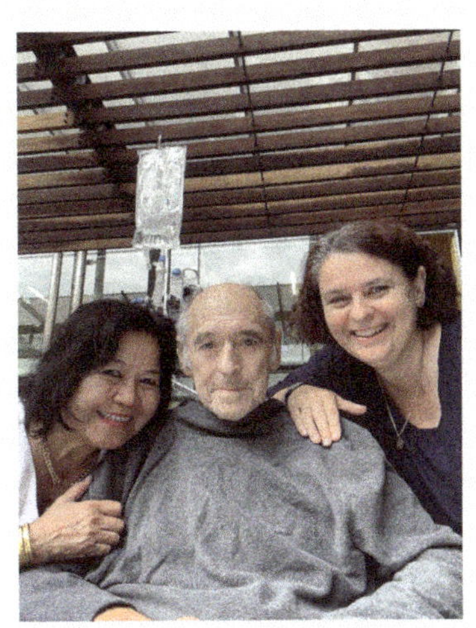

Venturing out of the hospital room for the first time after all Dad's surgeries

Despite my better judgement, I reasoned if anyone could beat the odds, it was Dad. I watched him fight his way back until he was well enough to be discharged. He was losing weight quickly, now a shadow of his former self. My focus was on juggling my work, study and placement commitments with all the visits to the hospital for both Mum and Dad. At this point I felt it was important to help Dad and Nang put together a will. This way everyone would have a clear sense of Dad's wishes and know what to expect if anything happened to him.

Mum was still having her treatments during Dad's admissions, and she was an amazing source of support despite her own struggles. It must have been so confronting for her to know Dad had such a poor prognosis. She told me it made her think: *My turn will come.* Mum's platelets were still not recovering, so she was booked for another scan. In the middle of dealing with Dad's illness and all the trips to the hospital, I was also attending all of Mum's oncology appointments. The most recent scan wasn't looking good with multiple areas of concern in her bones. The oncologist suggested this may represent metastatic disease to the bone, but since that's rare in ovarian cancer she wanted to do a bone marrow biopsy to rule out one of the secondary cancers Mum and I were afraid of (myelodysplastic disorders or leukaemia's).

Thankfully, Benni was very stable, being seizure free since July 2023, so Mum was able to support me by medicating Benni and looking after her when I was at the hospital visiting Dad. I was concerned Mum was going to need more care soon, particularly if there was metastatic bone cancer, as this can be very painful. I resolved to move Mum from the caravan park to my house, moving the business out to an external commercial rental so I could spend more time with Mum and look after her when she was sick. Dad's diagnosis had me thinking about mortality. I wanted to enjoy time with the important people in my life while they were still with me. Buddhist philosophy, quantum physics, and the intersection of science and spirituality always captivated me. I felt like I was trying to hold compassion wherever I could, no matter how difficult the situation or behaviour I may encounter. In my own mind, I was also trying to make sense of all of this. *What's the purpose of our existence anyway?*

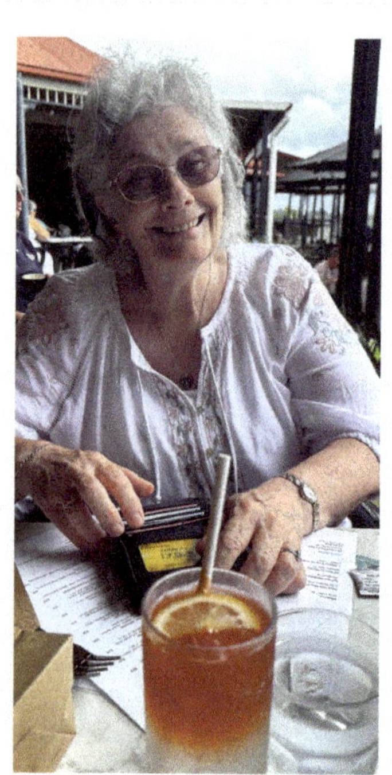

Spending quality time together after being told she likely has metastatic bone cancer

During one of Dad's many returns to the emergency department after discharge, he was very reflective. While waiting to be seen, and with tears, he looked directly at me and said, "What I did to your mum was unforgiveable. I understand why she chose to leave."

It was an admission I knew he wanted me to pass on to Mum, and I did so in good faith. Mum had been incredible while he was sick. She offered her perspective about cancer, visited him in hospital and promised him her easy chair so he would be more comfortable at home. It was always in

Mum's nature to be kind and compassionate, and she seemed to know that past hurts held little relevance at this time.

On November 15 Mum moved out of the caravan park and into my house in the little unit out front. The same day I moved my little business to an external rental in town. Dad was at home and too weak to be out and about but several people, including Nang, helped us facilitate this move for Mum, for which we were very grateful. Her easy chair went out to make Dad more comfortable, and we settled into our new living and my new working arrangements.

When Dad went home, he was supposed to be seen by the oncology team, but he still hadn't heard from them after more than a week. I noticed Dad was losing a lot of weight and, worried this was related to advancement of his cancer, I urged him to see the doctor. He was very optimistic. I believe he still felt he would beat his cancer. It was actually very hard to watch what felt to me like false hope grow. While I was always honest with him, it felt very lonely to be the only one giving him the bad news. I didn't want to be the one to squash any remaining hope. I decided it was my job to keep Dad updated with world news and all things quantum physics. He seemed interested, so I was trying to make things a bit lighter and more fun wherever I could. I'd share silly stories about things like the notion of how time isn't linear, we may all be living in a simulation, or the thought that aliens might actually be us but from a different dimension or time. In my view, he really enjoyed those little updates. He'd get a good laugh and I felt they were doing exactly what I hoped they would – ease any tension and lighten the mood.

He was in and out of hospital for ongoing issues with his weight and pain management. He was also approached about appointments to reverse his stoma, and fix his heart with a stent, all of which reinforced what felt like false hope. By early December, it was clear to me he was dying and his weight loss was likely cachexia (a syndrome that causes weight loss despite normal eating, usually associated with cancer). We needed to explore palliative care. After ongoing advocacy, Dad finally

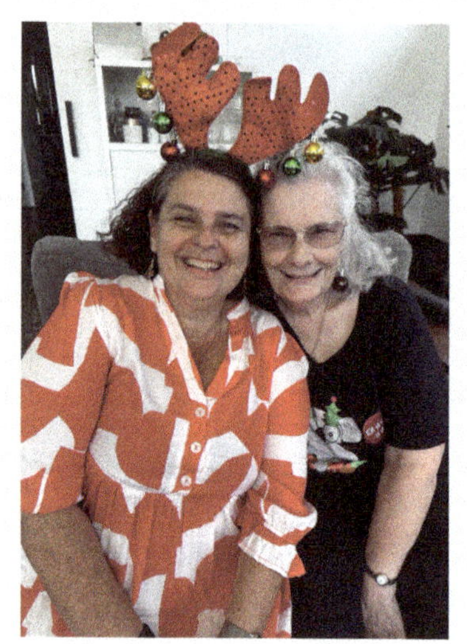

Mum and I at our mock Christmas

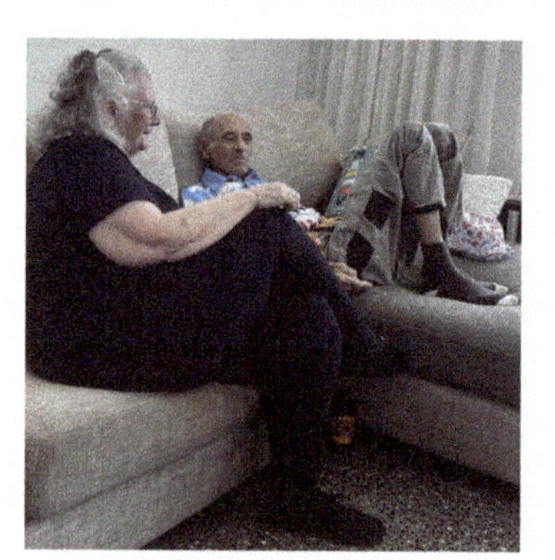

Mum and Dad at mock Christmas

got an appointment with a GP who referred him for urgent assessment with palliative care. On December 3, I attended Mum's palliative care appointment and I would be back on December 11 for Dad's. It was clear to me Dad wasn't likely to make it to Christmas. Mum was having her own challenges at this time, having her bone marrow biopsy on December 4 with results due on December 20.

After much consideration, I decided to talk to the family. I reasoned: *Maybe we need to think about having an earlier Christmas so he can be there.* In my mind, this was one of the hardest situations I could find myself in. I found it extremely difficult to get the words out any time I had to say out aloud, "I don't think he's going to make it to Christmas."

I couldn't believe how aggressive his cancer was. Dad was dying, and I sensed it would be sooner than people thought. From my point of view, I knew it was time to let people know what I felt I already knew.

We held a mock Christmas on December 7. Mum and Nang showed such grace in navigating this day. Ironically, Christmas was the one celebration Dad always hated but this time he played along, understanding the importance of the event for everyone else. I took some photos of my parents as I knew this would be my last opportunity to see them together and enjoying themselves. They reminisced about old times and created some amazing memories.

I'm so grateful for this special gathering, for the incredible grace and maturity of both Nang and Mum, and for the wonderful memories and photos I was able to take from this day. I knew the gravity of the pictures, as I knew both my parents would soon be gone. It was with a heavy heart and many tears that I reviewed these photos when I got home. Dad was given a date for his oncology appointment, December 20, the same date as Mum's appointment to see if her scan improved and get the results of her bone marrow biopsy. Great, two oncology appointments on the same day, only sadly I knew Dad wasn't going to make it to his.

As things progressed, I felt the need to take Dad back to hospital one last time so I could advocate for what I believed would help him, particularly stronger pain relief and palliative support. On December 17 the palliative care team took over his care. He still seemed resolute in the belief that he was going to "win" against his cancer. A member of the oncology team gently helped Dad to understand he wasn't going to recover. He finally understood that he was dying. Up until then, he was convinced he was going to beat the cancer. I always tried to be honest with him but some of the medical discussions seemed to be framed in softer or less direct terms. With Dad, who would always back himself for the win, this softer language, in my view, had the potential to leave things open to interpretation. He fought a great

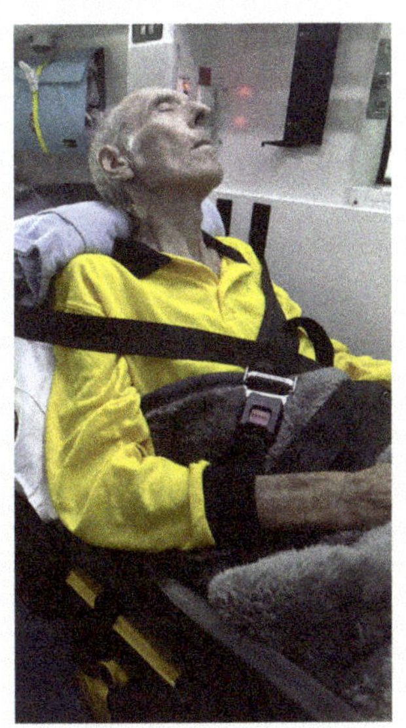

In the ambulance taking Dad back to hospital again

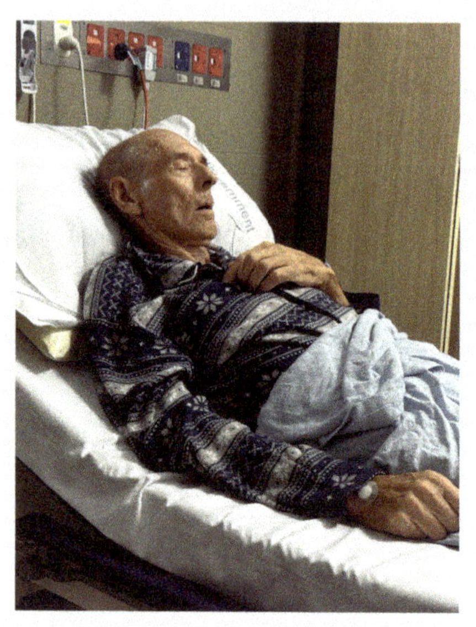

The final admission

fight, but he now knew he'd lost. He seemed defeated.

Dad expressed a desire not to die in hospital, and everyone wanted to honour Dad's wishes. I agreed to help make sure he could do this without being in pain. I felt confident in my ability to manage the medical aspects of his care as instructed, administer appropriate prescribed medications, and maintain a calm and supportive environment for both Dad and the people around him. I brought Benni in to visit Dad, and he did seem to enjoy having her there. She wasn't there for him – she was there for me. So many of these trips to the hospital were emotionally draining and for this one trip I at least was supported by the beautiful, ever-present Miss Benni.

Staying emotionally regulated had become somewhat of a superpower in such an emotionally charged environment. I felt this helped me navigate some difficult situations without getting personally involved or emotionally overwhelmed. Dad stayed in the hospital until the syringe pump for pain relief was set up, a plan for breakthrough medications made (additional medication for pain that breaks through the background infusion), and he was fully supported by the palliative care team on discharge. On December 19, Mum got to see Dad, resting in the comfy chair she had generously provided, for what would end up being the last time. These two people had spent over a quarter of a century together, through good and extremely bad times, experienced parenthood together, and were now sharing the challenging journey of a cancer diagnosis. Again, Nang was dignified, respecting this history and both their needs to connect at this time, allowing them precious time together, alone, to reminisce. Mum spoke to me about this time, mentioning that they didn't delve into much detail of their shared history, but she felt it was very generous of Nang. Although she said she would have appreciated a bit more time with him, their declining health didn't allow it. She was genuinely grateful for the time she did get to spend with Dad before he died.

The next day was Mum's big oncology appointment and would have also been Dad's but, as predicted, he was now on an end-of-life palliative care pathway. Mum's appointment felt strange to me. The results were described as inconclusive. The scan still showed multiple areas of concern in her bones. From what I understood, the plan was to continue her hormone therapy, continue to monitor her platelets and schedule a repeat scan in three months. Depending on the results, she would potentially have a bone biopsy from one of the more concerning areas. Between Mum's appointments, Dad's admissions to hospital, my business and the course, I was dizzy. I didn't know if I was Arthur or Martha! I was also really worried about what these results meant for Mum. I felt a sense of foreboding. On December 20, Dad took a turn for the worse and I knew this was the start of the dying process. By now I was on leave, had attended Mum's appointment, and was free to help with his medical management and pain relief. I sensed it was going to be a very difficult few days!

REST IN PEACE, DAD

No clothes nor possessions accompanied his entry into this world
His first foray into the unknown with seemingly endless hardship hurled
Then came family, there was no fortune nor fame
Just those who would eventually come to share his name
Many decades of adventure would follow, with no feat impossible to achieve
Until one day cancer came knocking, bringing suffering without reprieve
Though final days brought love, kindness and joy, with songs together sung
Deep in our hearts we knew all the while the end would certainly come
With his last words some calm relief, "No more worries, no more choices"
"We had a hell of a ride", "Yes, we did" uttered quivering voices
Before the night was over, before the rising of the sun
Like a thief under the cover of darkness, death would finally come
Now at peace in the vast expanse with the wind in his sails
No cares in this world, no rules, no judgements nor fails
May your compass point north and your soul be in flight
You can finally lay down your arms, Dad, you no longer need to fight
Rest easy on the ocean waves, there's no more work to do
As your every particle is returned to the sea,
this is how we will remember you

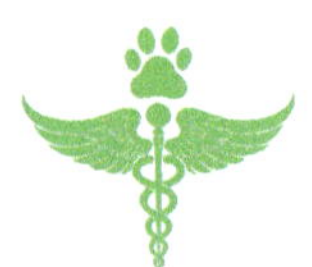

I packed a little bag as I didn't know how long I'd be gone, asked Mum if she could look after the dogs for me, and got in the car to head out to see Dad. I was listening to music on the way and heard Disturbed's version of the Simon & Garfunkel classic *The Sound of Silence*. I sobbed, belting out the song as loud as I could. There was so much history with Dad related to our extremely complex interpersonal dynamics. These were experiences that, for me, often involved feeling isolated and excluded. The line "Silence like a cancer grows" carried a lot of personal meaning.

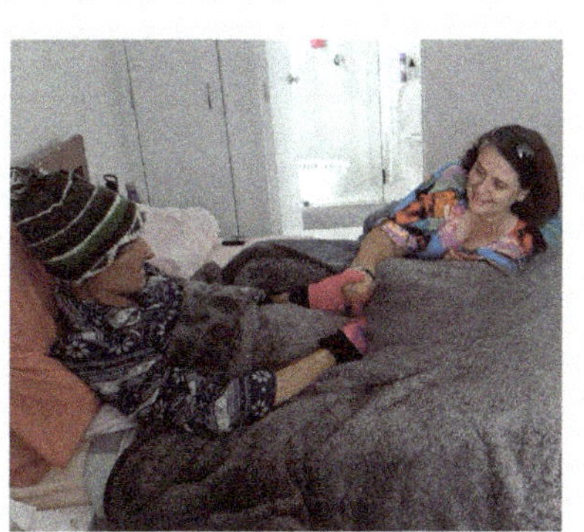

Dad with his beanie and gloves

I used to feel like my family was uniquely dysfunctional, but over time I've realised most families have their own version of complicated dynamics. From my perspective, tensions and old grievances can feel amplified at times of stress, particularly when someone comes into a large sum of money or when someone is gravely unwell. I have always felt that our family probably had more than its fair share of drama over the years, likely related to navigating Dad's difficult personality. As I drove, I thought about the weight of what I was about to experience and how important it would be for me to remain regulated, compassionate and self-aware. I would need all my new skills to get through this.

When I arrived, Dad was awake and interactive. Nang was tending to his needs. He was getting cold as his system was starting to shut down. He wore a beanie on his head and gloves on his hands to stay warm. The atmosphere felt tense and the air thick with grief in this little room. With ongoing problems with the hiccups, Dad was annoyed that once again this feature of his illness resurfaced. I felt the urge to fulfil my self-appointed role to bring some light to the situation.

I broke the silence with, "Dad, I heard a new version of *The Sound of Silence* on the way in. It's by a band called Disturbed. Have you heard it?"

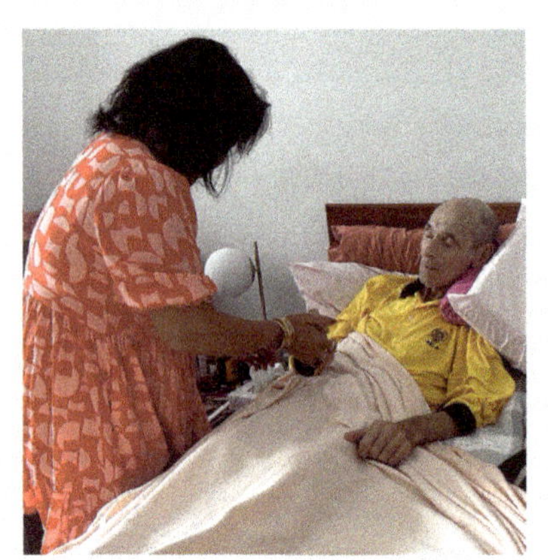

Nang caring for Dad

I knew how much he loved the original Simon and Garfunkel song and was surprised when he said, "Yes, it's beautiful."

I went on, figuring anything was better than sitting here in silence, waiting for the inevitable to happen. "I also listened to *The Gambler* on the way in. You used to love that song, Dad."

"I love Kenny Rogers."

Dad agreed it would be a lovely idea to play some music. Nang hunted around until she found a mobile speaker and I played *The Gambler* by Kenny Rogers from my phone. We all sang joyfully and clapped along to this song, including Dad. It was such a special moment. This song was really describing Dad's life and while carefully listening to the lyrics they took on a whole new meaning to me:

Son, I've made a life out of readin' people's faces
And knowin' what their cards were by the way they held their eyes

He had done just that in his life – made a living out of reading people and knowing when to walk away, knowing when to run! The song went on and we were all still clapping and singing along:

'Cause every hand's a winner and every hand's a loser
And the best that you can hope for is to die in your sleep

I tried to hold back the tears, but despite my best efforts they gently escaped my eyes and rolled down my cheeks. I thought: *This is what lasting memories are made of. I will remember this moment for the rest of my life.*

We played music, clapped, sang and cried together, with Dad slipping in and out of consciousness while I assisted with administering any necessary prescribed medications through the line inserted by the palliative care nurse. The background infusions for agitation, nausea, pain relief and the terrible intractable hiccups were also ticking away. One of his all-time favourites was the John Denver song *Country Road*. When this song came on, Dad became quite alert again and started clapping and loudly singing along. Nang took some footage of this moment to capture the joy and sorrow, and document such a treasured memory. As he sang along, one hand in Nang's, I felt he was remembering all his amazing adventures.

He looked deeply in Nang's eyes, mustered all his energy and sang louder, "... take me home, to the place I belong, West Virginia, mountain mama, take me home, country roads!"

Eventually the music was turned down and then off to allow him to sleep. Music would become a valuable distraction, providing much-needed respite from the weight of this situation.

Dad was still in and out of consciousness. I tried to have little naps in between but very little sleep came. We didn't want Dad to be in pain and I personally felt the weight of the responsibility heavily, so I was up and down all night. The air felt thick with grief, the room dark and quiet, apart from occasional sobbing. There seemed to be a lot of questions, and at the time I felt like I was the only person around Dad who had experience with death and the dying process. I believe my medical knowledge helped me to keep everyone as informed and reassured as I could. I was really missing Benni, wishing she could be here with me, but knowing this wasn't the appropriate environment for her. I needed to minimise her stress. The last thing I needed right now was for Benni to have a seizure. I knew she would be safe, well cared for and happy with Mum.

When the nurse came in the morning, I established Dad was stable enough for me to duck home, get a few things, and see Mum and Benni. I felt a palpable sense of relief leaving that little room. Although I saw it as an incredible privilege to be involved, it also felt like an emotional pressure cooker. While there always seemed to be complex relationships and a lot of history with the people who surrounded Dad, from my perspective, now was a time to set aside all differences, focus fully on caring for Dad, and provide much-needed support for those around me, particularly Nang, who seemed very distraught, and Mum, who was in a battle of her own. Staying true to my values of peace and compassion throughout this experience was my priority.

I grabbed a quick shower, debriefed with Mum about Dad's condition, and laid down to have a quick nap. Benni could tell I was upset. She laid right next to me with some part of her body always in contact. She snuggled in, giving me a classic Benni cuddle as I twirled her soft ears and cried. *Thank God for the dog* echoed in my head. I quickly realised I was never going to get any sleep. I packed a little bag, including a travel neck pillow for Dad, as I'd noticed how uncomfortable he was, gave Benni one more hug, and called Nang to check in and let her know I was headed back. It was an easy 25-minute drive, but I knew this time I wouldn't be coming home again until he had passed, so it was an emotional trip. A few minutes before I arrived, I gathered my emotions and took time to regulate. *Here we go.*

Dad was much less alert this day and there were many more times where it felt appropriate to remain respectfully quiet and allow him to rest. I was also exhausted so I tried to grab some rest where I could in between administering medications. A few people came to see Dad and once again I felt Nang was respectful, demonstrating grace and compassion, allowing each of them valuable time to say goodbye. At times, I would look at Dad and find it very difficult to reconcile my memories of a man who had been aggressive and frightening in my childhood with the vulnerable old man in front of me. I deeply appreciated the privilege of being able to care for him at this time.

I also came to the cathartic realisation that I was different from my dad because I still held compassion for a man who had shown very little for me. I spent my whole life wanting to be different to him. I wanted to be tolerant, compassionate, loving, kind and fair. In this moment, I realised I had succeeded. This was a deep realisation, and it gave me some additional peace, closure and some self-compassion. My relationship with Dad was the most difficult relationship in my life but I had managed to redefine it, coming to a place of deep peace with him. There was no blame. No anger. No forgiveness required. I accepted him, fully, just the way he was, and I now offered myself this same acceptance. I believe accepting someone exactly how they are, without willing them to change, is one of the greatest gifts you can give someone. Dad's life was difficult and filled with many challenges. He made many mistakes, hurt many people, but he was human and deserved love and compassion as much as anyone else.

At one point that day, I was on my own with Dad, which in my recollection was uncommon. In a moment of lucidity, he took my hand and said, "We had a hell of a ride, didn't we?"

"Yes we did, Dad."

Nang entered the room not long after, took his other hand, and he looked directly at me, gently placing my hand on Nang's. His eyes communicated desperation as he could no longer speak but I felt I knew exactly what he was saying. "I'll take care of her, Dad. I promise."

We had agreed it was important to take photos and videos to remember the special little moments. This was such a special and lasting moment I took the opportunity to take a photo, so we had a tangible memory to look back on. Appearing relieved, he nodded and drifted back off to sleep as a tear rolled down my cheek. These lucid moments were few and far between now and so very special. Later that evening, close to midnight, it all started to hit Nang. She started to cry and hugged Dad tightly, but he was unconscious and unresponsive. She began to wail. This was the same wail I heard in medicine when women lost their babies. It pierced the silence and created a sensation of tight discomfort in my chest.

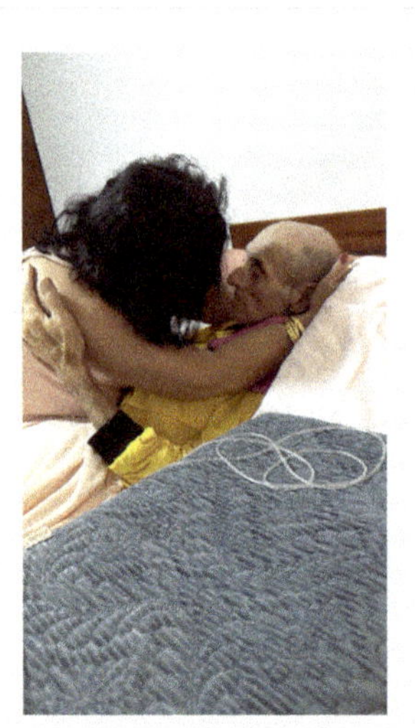

Dad miraculously awakening to console Nang

She seemed absolutely grief stricken and there was nothing anyone could do to console her. She kept crying, "Why? Why do you have to leave me?"

And just like a fairy tale, Dad woke up and gave her a huge hug, patting her gently on the back, consoling her the way only her partner could in that moment. But this was no fairy tale. Tears again escaped from my eyes. I could only imagine the heartbreak of watching your partner of 30 years dying in front of you, and Dad's heartbreak knowing he couldn't relieve her of her grief. He was dying and there was nothing he could do but accept it. This was the last of Dad's lucid moments.

It had been a rough night for me. I was exhausted. Dad required a lot of breakthrough medication overnight, so the palliative care team was notified. When they arrived to review him, I communicated that

Dad seemed to have increased breakthrough pain relief requirements, and after review, they increased the infusion. I asked quietly, "What do you want me to do with the pump when he passes?" She demonstrated how to turn off the pump and advised to ring them any time if needed. I took aside the lovely nurse for a quiet conversation.

"His breathing pattern has changed again and I think he may pass overnight. Can you please leave us with some more breakthrough medication?" I asked.

"Absolutely," she replied. "We will make sure you have everything you need."

The beautiful palliative care team left plenty of breakthrough medications and made sure the increased background infusion was effective before they left. They also provided some updates, taking some of the pressure I felt off me to relay the medical aspects of his care. Understandably, there seemed to be a constant stream of questions, but I feel I did my best to calmly relay accurate information. Having this medicalised role was helpful in keeping me focused on emotional regulation and it made me feel useful in what felt like an incredibly disempowering situation.

However, I have to admit there were times when it also weighed on me, with the tension putting a strain on my ability to cope. With Dad's deteriorating state, I didn't feel like I could leave so I could talk to Mum only over the phone, calling and texting where possible. I was worried about her and Benni and remained cautious about not oversharing with Mum. She was his wife of 25 years, my mother and was in the middle of facing her own mortality. I felt it was very important at this time to hold compassion for Mum. Benni wasn't showing any signs of distress, thank goodness. Mum was doing a great job of taking care of her, and I'm sure Benni was taking care of Mum as well.

Around 8:30pm, Dad's breathing pattern seemed to change again. From my knowledge of the dying process, I felt this was the final breathing pattern. While it was still intermittent, I felt it was important to make it clear to Nang that if she wanted to be in the room when Dad passed, it would be advisable not to leave the room from now on. The need for breakthrough medications seemed to diminish and we settled in, swapping positions within the room from on the bed next to Dad to a chair next to the bed. I was lying next to him when around 12.15am on December 23, he took one last, loud, deep breath.

Nang said, "Oh God, this is it, isn't it?" I reached over and put my palm on his now skeletal, cold chest in time to feel his heart stop beating under my warm hand. Tears escaped my eyes as I focused on the task of confirming his passing.

After waiting about 30 seconds I confirmed, "Yes, Nang, he's gone."

Dad passed peacefully, surrounded by love and care, and pain free, as promised, at 12.15am on December 23, 2024 at 80 years of age. As if part of a sacred, silent contract between us, we stayed with him until the very end.

I turned off the pump and called the palliative care team. Everyone who needed to be notified was advised of his passing. The palliative care nurse attended to formally confirm his death and, once Dad was dressed, there was nothing left to do but wait for the funeral director to collect him. I packed up, rang Mum to tell her I was on my way home and left. I felt such a relief to leave that little room. I felt deeply privileged to have been involved in Dad's care but I wasn't in my home, so it was an uncomfortable environment for me. I was missing all my puppy support and the sense of safety my home provided. I was finally home and, after debriefing with Mum, I fell into my bed sobbing, cuddling Benni and trying to process the events of the past few days. The experience had given me some incredible gifts. Sometimes the best gifts come not from good times but through hardship and deep self-reflection. I was back in my beautiful home, my peaceful, safe place, with my beautiful Benni and my incredible mum who had shown grace and dignity throughout this experience despite the incredible battle she was having herself.

I was so tired and spent from my personal cognitive, emotional load and sleep deprivation of those few days. Mum was also exhausted, so we decided to stay home on Christmas Day despite previous invites to gatherings. I was very emotional and cried every hour or so without warning, so I was very grateful to have made and stuck to this decision. I needed to be in my safe haven, surrounded by my supports and self-care. This time was incredibly difficult for me and in times of stress like this, I previously had difficulty maintaining my calm. Thankfully, I noticed I didn't respond the same way to external challenges anymore. Through devout Buddhist practice, including meditation and radical compassion, I was able to navigate this period without turning on myself, the way I had done so many times before in the face of loss or external stressors. I rooted myself firmly in the belief that we are all equal humans, using the tools we have available to us at the time to navigate life the best way we know how.

I could put my hand on my heart and know that throughout Dad's illness, death and aftermath, I felt I had been honest, respectful, supportive, loving and compassionate. This was all that mattered to me because the fact is that was all I had control over. In my opinion, living true to your values is deeply protective. No matter how negative any external situation or rhetoric seems, if you know deep within yourself that you were true to your values, you can sleep at night and not internalise external stressors or what others say or think about you. After all, external situations and opinions are out of your control anyway so worrying about them is futile.

Mum was my only external source of support at this time and I was very grateful, but providing this support seemed to take its toll on her health. We talked deeply about how people react to stress in life and despite how unwell she was, Mum expressed how she still felt the need to hold compassion for others, including Dad. It's a value we shared. Ultimately, she got to decide how much she let external life challenges disrupt her peace. She had a battle of her own to fight and our conversations seemed to give her some solace.

Other than a few little things, Mum and I agreed the only thing we wanted from each other for Christmas was time. Time can't be bought or sold, and you can't get it back when it's gone. In the spirit of valuing our time together, we bought a spa day voucher. On January 4, 2025, we went for an almost-all-day spa that included treatments, lunch together and time to create some beautiful memories in a calm, supportive and relaxing environment. If the past few months had taught me anything, it was to value the time you have with the people you love.

Time is a curious thing. We take it for granted, and we tend to give a lot of time and attention to things and people who cause us grief. One of the methods we use in dog training is to give attention and time to the behaviours we want, and ignore the ones we don't want. I made a promise to myself after Dad's death to work on spending more of my time and energy with the people who cared about me and treated me well, making sure they knew how much I loved and cared for them too, and spend less time and energy on the people who I perceived to be unkind or uncaring. I reasoned, you get more of what you put your focus on!

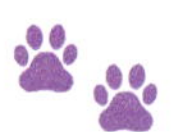

On Monday February 3, 2025, Dad's ashes were spread on a local beach near his favourite lighthouse. A fitting place for such an adventurous soul who lived many of his 80 years on or in the water. I wrote a poem for Dad and brought my jade prayer beads along so I could radiate compassion and love. I said my goodbyes and went back to check on Mum, who couldn't attend. Her situation was very uncertain. We were still waiting for a repeat scan to see what to do next. She seemed very nervous and so was I.

Grief is a funny thing. It comes when it wants to, not when it's invited. I needed to let it be there when it came. I allowed myself to cry and to think about Dad and our years together. I thought about the good times and the bad, and honoured his memory wherever I could. I felt like I had a very good understanding of how his life circumstances impacted on him and how that in turn affected his behaviour. I accepted him warts and all, and this made the grieving process a little easier I think.

I'VE GOT YOU

"I've got you, Mum, I'm here for you through thick and thin"
I whisper as I wait with you, aware of the distinct hospital din
The machines, drips and equipment interrupt any moments of peace
I gently brush your hair, waiting for someone to make the pain cease
Each time a little bit of hope seems to emerge, it's snatched away again
As the sands beneath your feet begin to shift, once more returns the pain
An ostensibly relentless battle for just a little bit of control
Ends in disempowerment, as I grapple with the
reality your loss will leave a huge hole
The battle has been long and hard, with ground won and lost along the way
You fought so gallantly, even knowing cancer would probably win one day
So much pain you suffered in this life from those
you should have been able to trust
Those days are over now, no need to even give
a thought to those who were unjust
I want you to know, before you leave this world,
my life was better because you were here
The girls and I will miss you so much, we will shed more than the odd tear
However, most will be tears of joy for the
wonderful memories we have shared
Despite the tenacity you gave me as your
daughter, I'm still feeling unprepared
I will draw on the lessons I've learnt watching
your incredible strength and grace
I know we'll meet again on the other side of the
rainbow bridge, I'll look for your friendly face
For now, it's back into the ring we go for the
last battles, round four, round five
I've got you, Mum, until your very last breath, you will find me by your side

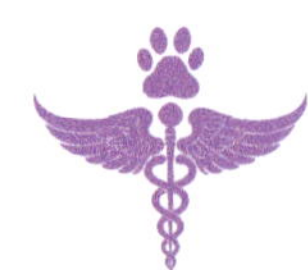

Things seemed to settle down for a while, and I was able to get back to some form of normalcy. I was still grieving but functional and back at work. While the dog training course was ongoing, I was feeling a bit behind from the time away while Dad was sick. I was finally able to get back on track, completing the rest of the basic assessments by early March. I was also able to complete many of my placement hours, so it felt like I was completely back on track. I hadn't been able to complete the course in six months as intended, but I was still well within the 12-month timeframe. I completed all the written components and started looking at the requirements for the practical assessments.

My schedule was busy and Mum's repeat scan looked much the same. There was an ongoing concern that Mum had metastatic disease in her bones, with a bone biopsy booked for March 27. I researched metastatic bone cancer and, while this wasn't a great thing to have, you could still live several years with appropriate treatment. Consequently, I felt optimistic Mum would be able to get the treatment she needed to survive and potentially for several years.

One night when I came home from work, Mum mentioned she was feeling short of breath during the day. I asked a few questions but reasoned that due to her low cell counts she may be anaemic. Still, I tried to convince her to go to the GP, reminding her of the possible serious complications like blood clots in the lungs. No matter what I said to Mum, she was adamant she didn't want to see the doctor just yet. She had an appointment the following week to have her bone biopsy, with blood tests due a few days before. She absolutely refused to go to the GP any earlier. The next day, I decided to spend some time with her to see if I could witness this shortness of breath as she walked around the house. Mum was significantly short of breath, easily fatigued and clearly unwell. This time, I used stronger language and urged her to go to the doctor, but she still refused. I had back-to-back clients all afternoon until 6pm, but I was very concerned about leaving her alone. I called between clients a couple of times to check in on her but she was quite annoyed with me, saying, "Stop calling, Jo, everything's fine. I'll talk to you when you get home!"

When I arrived home, I went straight out the front to check on Mum, only to find her packing a bag. She said, "You'll be proud of me. I went and had some blood tests done and they just called to say I need to go in." As a retired doctor, I wanted to know what the results of these blood tests were but she couldn't tell me. Instead, she called the oncology doctor so I could speak to them myself. The doctor didn't tell me much, other than to say her blood tests were quite abnormal. They were concerned about a pulmonary embolism (blood clot in the lungs) but there may also be some other kind of complication going on. They needed to bring her in for further investigation.

We spent several hours in the emergency department, waiting for test after test. A scan excluded a pulmonary embolism and Mum was still waiting for some other blood tests to come back. I decided I needed to duck home and check on the dogs, medicate Benni and bring back some essentials for Mum in case she was admitted. At this stage, I was still quite convinced this was some kind of complication related to her cancer. *But what could it be if it's not a pulmonary embolism?* I knew you could get some fairly serious complications associated with bone cancer but I didn't want to speculate.

I wasn't expecting what happened next. Mum's blood tests came back positive for a condition called disseminated intravascular coagulation (DIC). This was a serious complication, but it was one I was most familiar with in association with sepsis, not cancer. In DIC, there's an impairment to the normal clotting cascade, causing either excessive clotting or excessive bleeding. I was a bit baffled as to why Mum would have this condition, as she didn't have an infection. When the doctor told us they thought she may have leukaemia, I was devastated. This really did feel like the worst-case scenario. On March 13, 2025 only three months after losing Dad, here I was again in a hospital emergency department receiving a devastating diagnosis for someone I loved.

To confirm this diagnosis, Mum would have to have a bone marrow biopsy again. We notified all the relevant family members and they did the bone marrow biopsy to confirm the doctor's suspicions.

In a tiny little corner of the hospital, a lovely doctor sat us down, asking Mum, "Has someone explained what's going on to you yet, Susanne?"

"Yes, I have DIC," Mum replied confidently.

"Okay, great. Well, DIC is a dangerous condition. It can be hard to treat. I think that what's causing it may be a blood cancer called acute myeloid leukaemia (AML). Do you know what that is?"

"Yes, my daughter's a doctor so I know about leukaemia." She gestured towards me.

He continued, "Unfortunately, this is a nasty blood cancer and when you get it after chemotherapy it can be very hard to treat and doesn't usually respond well to treatment anyway."

I could see Mum trying to process the information. She understood the gravity of the diagnosis and we had discussed this possibility before.

"How long do you think I have?" she enquired, sounding defeated.

"Untreated, the prognosis is really poor. So sorry," he said softly as he passed Mum some tissues.

"I need to know how long?" Mum pressed for an answer

The doctors looked at one another, understandably reluctant to commit to a timeframe, but Mum was insistent. Eventually they confirmed her worst fears. She was unlikely to survive the week without treatment.

I was numb. *How could this be happening?* Mum remained calm and composed as she always did. Then we sat and talked about what to do next. They were treating her DIC, having discussed treatment for leukaemia and the low chances of success.

A cancer warrior to the end, Mum told the doctors, "I want to fight while I still have fight left in me." They talked about the treatment options for leukaemia in more detail. Mum agreed she would like to give at least one round of treatment a go. The doctors, while very supportive, were clear she still may not survive the week or the treatment and the likelihood of this secondary cancer responding to treatment was very low. After they left, Mum and I took a photo with our tongues out in defiance. Mum jokingly referred to it as her "fuck cancer" photo.

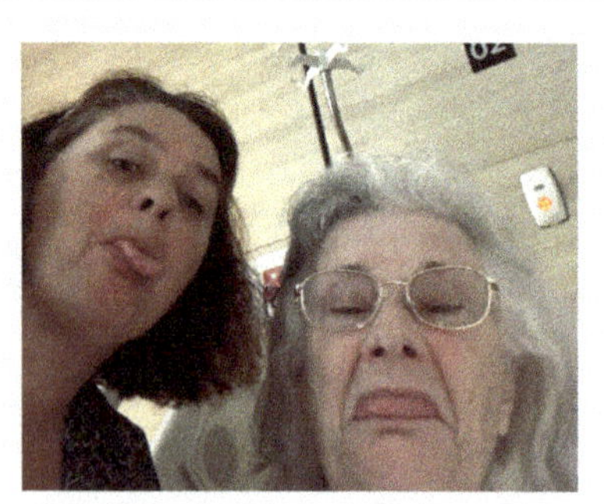

A moment of defiance the day she was diagnosed with AML

I set about contacting everyone Mum asked me to, letting them know they should probably come and see her while they could. Perhaps most importantly for Mum, I also contacted her sister, my aunty (who I affectionately call Aunty K), in New South Wales and advised her to come up as soon as she could. The hospital initially denied access for Bella due to the nature of the ward where Mum was. After several hours of advocacy, Mum was finally moved to a ward where she could see her beloved girl. I was exhausted from the fight but so relieved when I walked Bella in to see her. My heart was breaking as I watched them interact, knowing Bella and I would be losing Mum soon. When I took Bella home, I fell into Benni's loving embrace as she tilted her head from side to side, trying to figure out why I was so upset. She didn't hesitate to give me her full attention and unconditional love. *Thank God for this dog!*

Some family came to visit, including Aunty K. Mum stayed in hospital having the treatment, which she said was better than the chemotherapy. Ironically, we were told the chemotherapy used to reduce her chance of worsening peripheral neuropathy, can sometimes be associated with the development of blood cancers like AML. She responded well to her initial DIC treatment and started on the first round of therapy for AML. She got to come home on day pass for a family lunch on March 15 and proudly brought home with her a sparkling red wheelie walker.

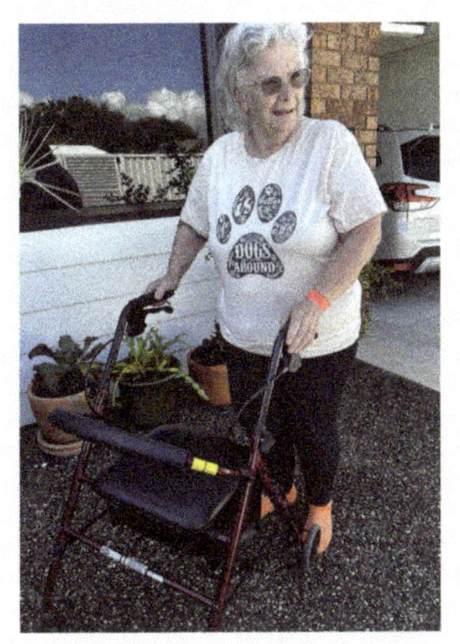

"I told you I'd get my wheelie walker one day!"

As she got out of the car, she made me take a photo of her, saying, "I told you I'd get my wheelie walker one day!" She was always trying to lighten the mood.

Aunty K and I had cooked a roast, and several family members who were around at the time joined us. It was a lovely, relaxed outing but it did exhaust her. Just before she was due to go back to the hospital, she asked us to go into her bedroom. She spoke at length about her wishes once she was gone, shared loving words, and talked frankly about how hard this journey had been for her. She talked about her values of forgiveness and compassion, and asked that we take care of each other.

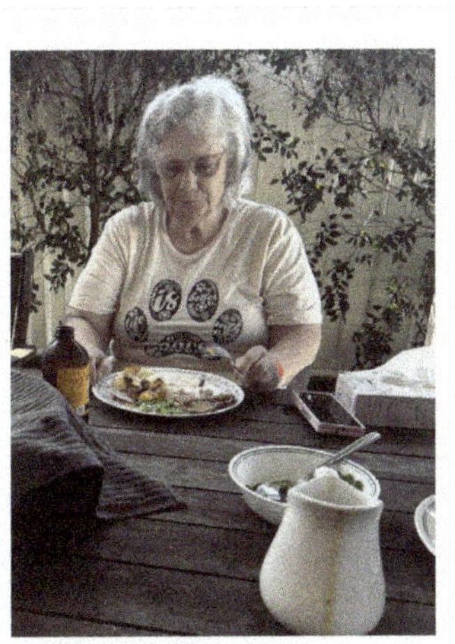

Our last roast dinner together

Mum was having injections, as well as blood, platelet and other transfusions, every other day at the hospital, and blood tests in between. She was a walking pharmacy of pills and absolutely covered in bruises. Every time someone came in they wanted to put a needle into her. I asked them if they could put in a PICC (peripherally inserted central catheter – a line that stays in so you don't have to keep having injections) but they were reluctant to do this because of the risk of infection. Mum was complaining of being a pin cushion, so Aunty K made her a voodoo doll out of hospital gloves and stuffed it with a hand towel. I brought her one pin and she was off. She had the whole ward laughing about her little voodoo doll.

"I'll get it in first time, I promise," they would say.

I was cancelling every appointment and commitment, knowing my beautiful clients would understand. Most of them knew and loved Mum or had heard my funny little stories about her. Bella was staying in the front unit of my house (where Mum lived) with Aunty K and her dog, Molly, but every time I saw Bella I felt so sad for her. I knew she would soon be without her precious someone and the realisation broke my heart.

Towards the end of March, Mum stabilised enough to go home and once she was settled Aunty K also went home and waited to be called back. The doctors weren't sure how long the treatment would give Mum, but she seemed to be responding so they thought she may get a few months out of it if she was lucky. She eventually had a PICC line inserted and was having treatment and infusions as an outpatient every couple of days. It was a gruelling schedule – she was exhausted by it but happy to be home. They arranged for some other equipment to be sent to the house, so we had what we needed to care for Mum if her condition deteriorated quickly.

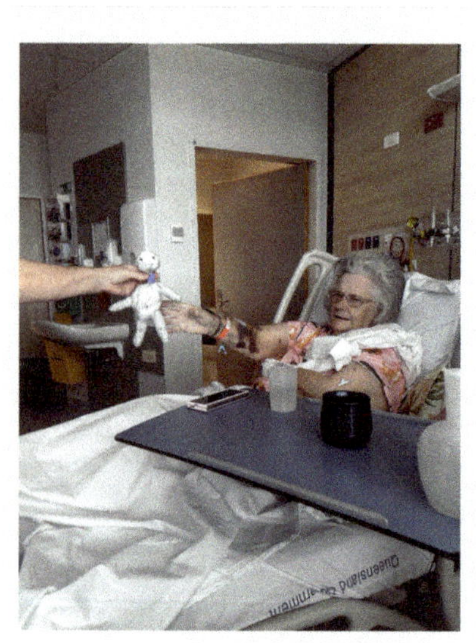

Aunty K handing Mum her voodoo doll

I remember Mum saying to me, "It would be okay, Jodi, if I felt like I was dying, but I just don't."

She was having a very hard time coming to terms with the fact she was dying and still felt so very much alive.

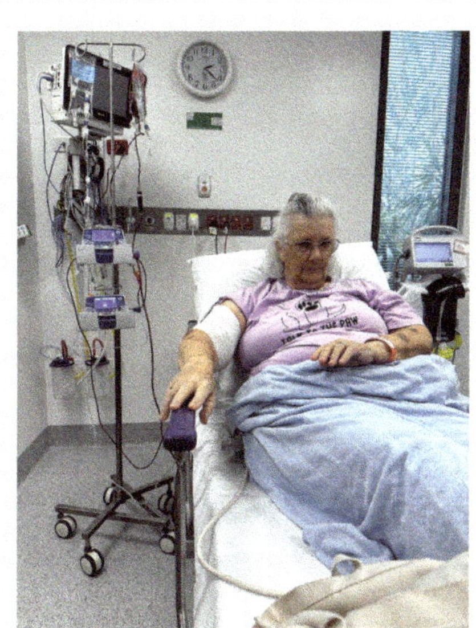

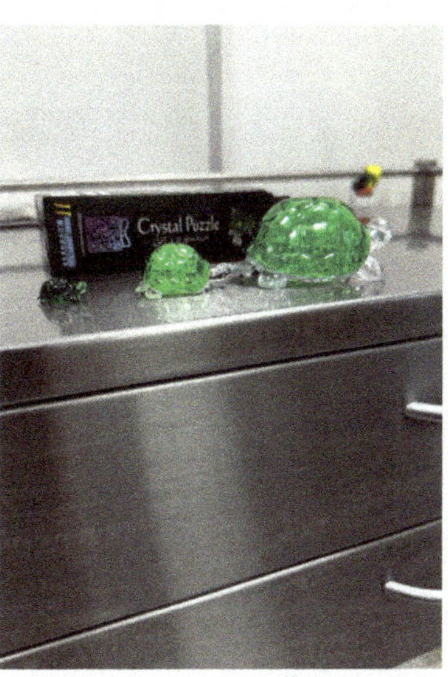

One of many blood transfusions while we made our little turtles

On April 4 we went to the hospital as usual to have her treatment, blood and platelets. This was the last appointment before her scheduled bone marrow biopsy to see if the treatment was working. This time I brought the 3D puzzle of three little green turtles Mum gifted me for Christmas. I figured now was as good a time as any to put them together. We sat reading and misinterpreting instructions, fumbling and dropping pieces, giggling quietly at our ineptitude until all three little turtles were proudly together. This was another one of those moments that will stay with me forever. We passed the hours while her infusions were running, we laughed and just spent precious time together.

On April 6, the weekend before her bone marrow biopsy, we went to a spiritual church together, just as we had done all those years ago at Eagle Lodge. Mum was pale, weak and tired but she was adamant we do this together. We enjoyed brunch first at a local café then drove up to the church to have a look. We were never church-going people, but I was becoming more interested in finding others with similar Buddhist philosophies nearby. With this in mind, Mum found this little spiritual church she said she wanted to go and look at with me. We laughed at how nervous we had been at Eagle Lodge, reminisced about what a lovely time it was in our lives and how this time we really hoped these people hugged us! They welcomed us with open arms, but it was no Eagle Lodge. We stayed for a while until I could see Mum was struggling and we drove back home. The car ride was one story after another about the positive living course, Eagle Lodge, the STEPS course, the time on the boat and all the lovely memories we shared.

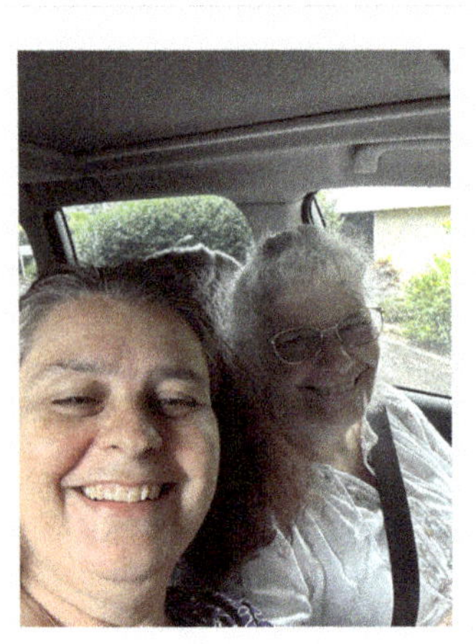

Coming home from the spiritual church

April 7 was bone marrow biopsy day. Soon we would find out if the treatment would buy her any more time. We arrived for her appointment at 8.30am and waited for hours for her to go in for the biopsy, finally going in at around midday. I waited for her to get back, but it took longer than I thought. I was starting to get worried when they finally wheeled her back in. She was in a lot of pain and as the minutes ticked by this got gradually worse. At 2pm, they moved her to the emergency department where she waited for a scan. It seemed to take forever. I knew she had low platelets, which made her higher risk for bleeding complications. From my medical background I also understood, because of how deep a bone marrow biopsy is, a lot of blood could potentially be lost before it became visible. She said they took two attempts and it only increased my worry that she may have a bleed.

After waiting for a while she seemed stable, so at 7pm I couldn't wait any longer – Benni needed her medication at home. I managed to race home to medicate and feed the dogs. While I was getting in the car to come back, I got a call from a nurse, informing me Mum had deteriorated and was being taken to theatre. I was able to talk to Mum for a second, and she sounded worried. I told her she was in good hands, the dogs were fine and I was on my way back in. Once again, I found myself sitting in an empty hospital at night, waiting for someone I loved to come out of a serious operation. They rang me when she was in recovery and let me know I could come up and see her and get a brief update. I spoke to her doctor who explained she had a major bleed from an artery that was thought to have been damaged during the biopsy, a potential complication we were made aware of before the procedure. Controlling the bleeding had been difficult, so they needed to ligate (tie off) the artery. I sensed how lucky she was to have survived this.

I hugged her tight, and whispered, "I love you, Mum," before finally leaving the hospital and getting home close to midnight. What a day!

Mum stayed in hospital waiting for things to settle, waiting for the results of her biopsy. Visits from Bella were the highlight of Mum's days when she was in hospital. I tried to make sure I brought Bella in as much as I could. She was a form of medicine Mum couldn't get anywhere else. Benni was my medicine, and I spent as much time with her and Freya as I could when I wasn't at the hospital. Mum developed a condition called tumour lysis syndrome, which occurs as the result of a build-up of toxins from dying cancer cells during treatment. She was now being treated for this and having her platelets and blood replaced. She then developed an infection, which, given the severity of her illness and what she had just been through, came as no surprise. However, with AML, the doctors advised that infections for Mum could be life-threatening.

They started her on some antibiotics. While the nurse was talking to her, I overheard the medical team reporting how Mum still had a very high blast count in her peripheral blood. In doctor speak, I understood this to mean the treatment wasn't working. The team advised we would have to wait for the formal results of the biopsy but, in my view, this and the infection were very bad news.

On April 10, I was heading into the hospital so I could be there when the doctor came to see Mum. We were expecting to get the formal results of the bone marrow biopsy. I called while I was on my way to check in. Mum wanted to wait for me to get there. She said she didn't understand the results. However, when I arrived, it was obvious Mum had been crying. She understood the results but wanted to tell me in person rather than over the phone.

"Sit down, Jo," she said as she patted the edge of the bed gently. "The treatment hasn't worked and there's nothing more they can do. I want you to be strong. You're not allowed to cry or you'll start me up again."

I held her hand and squeezed gently. "Fucking hell, Mum, that sucks!" It's unusual for me to swear but what else could I say? I stepped away to control my tears.

"I know, you're telling me!" she retorted.

I stayed as composed as I could as she asked me if I would help her tell others and I agreed. The doctors came back in and explained the findings of the biopsy – there had been virtually no response to treatment. While the decision would always be up to Mum, more treatment wouldn't usually be recommended. Mum's wonderful regular oncologist, who had been keeping an eye on her the whole time, came to see her. We said our goodbyes to this amazing clinician who had taken extraordinarily good care of my mum over the past three years. Mum requested the treating teams discuss the results and options again with me present to help both of us understand what we were facing. The medical staff were so supportive and always made sure she was well informed, affording Mum much-valued autonomy around her decisions. Mum took in all the information and made the awful decision to stop treatment and go home.

I promised Mum I would be with her from the beginning of this cancer journey to the very end, and I would ensure she didn't have any unnecessary pain. She chose to die at home, in my little unit out the front of our little house near the beach. I contacted my Aunty K and told her it was time. She hopped in the car with my mum's 94-year-old mother and made her way up. I tried to find somewhere Nana could stay so Aunty K could help me care for Mum while she was dying, but no-one seemed to be able to accommodate her at short notice. I rang Nang who was on her way back from a visit to the boat in New Zealand. When she agreed to look after Nana, I breathed a sigh of relief. I decided to accommodate them in a motel nearby.

Once again, I felt Nang showed grace in a very difficult situation. She knew Nana from her time with Dad. They always seemed to get along well and Nang didn't seem to mind taking care of Nana. I was very grateful Nang would do this for Mum, and I know Mum really appreciated it. Mum had suffered so much in her life. I wanted her to feel safe now and I would need Aunty K's support to care for her. Aunty K, her beautiful little dog, Molly, and Nana arrived on the evening of April 12, seeing Mum briefly at the hospital before checking in to the motel. Nang arrived a few days later.

Mum decided she wanted to have another family get-together when she got home. On April 15 we finally got to bring Mum home. She was welcomed with her favourite wheelie walker and helped inside. We spent time sitting, talking and laughing about silly things. Having Aunty K there was such a relief. She was making sure we enjoyed some light moments, just as Mum would have wanted. We also talked about logistics.

"What do you think will take me?" Mum wanted to know what I thought would most likely cause her death.

"Remember the doctors said the most common cause of death in AML is infection."

"I don't want to be in pain," she said. I reassured her I would ensure she had all the pain relief she needed.

"You have to promise me you'll let Bella say goodbye. I don't want her to think I just left her."

"I'll make sure she stays with you, Mum," I said as tears started to fall gently down my cheeks.

"Thank you. I just couldn't stand her thinking I left her."

"I promise I'll take good care of her, Mum. Benni will too."

"I know," Mum said, sobbing.

The other dogs would also need to know Gran (what the dogs "called" Mum) had gone as well. She showed me where all her important paperwork was and instructed me on what to do with everything. One of the beautiful things about my relationship with Mum is how we could talk about anything openly and honestly. We'd already worked through all our past issues, said everything we wanted – good and bad – and it was a lovely place to be. There was nothing left unsaid or undone in our relationship. I made sure she knew, while she was alive and well, how much she meant to me. She told me how much she loved me, was never afraid to be honest with me, and had been an incredible source of support for at least the past decade of my life, showing me what I meant to her each day. This was the most restorative relationship.

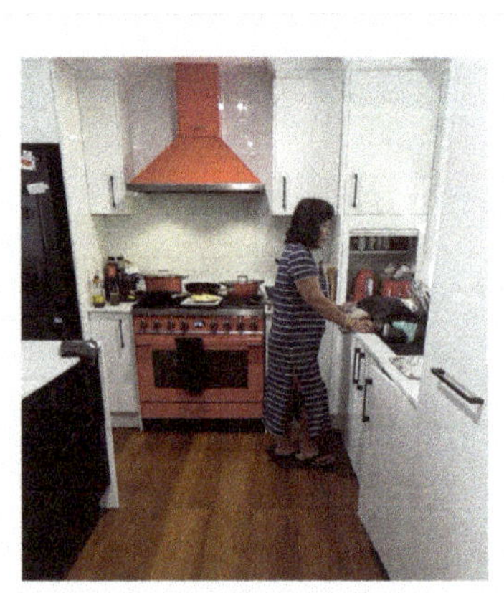

Nang helping out, April 17

On April 17 we hosted a beautiful family brunch with those who could attend, including Nang who was looking after Nana. This felt like the very special moments I experienced with Dad before he died. Mum looked so well, she interacted with some of her beautiful extended family, ate with us, rested in between interactions, laughed and spent valuable hours with the family. This was such a peaceful, serene, positive and

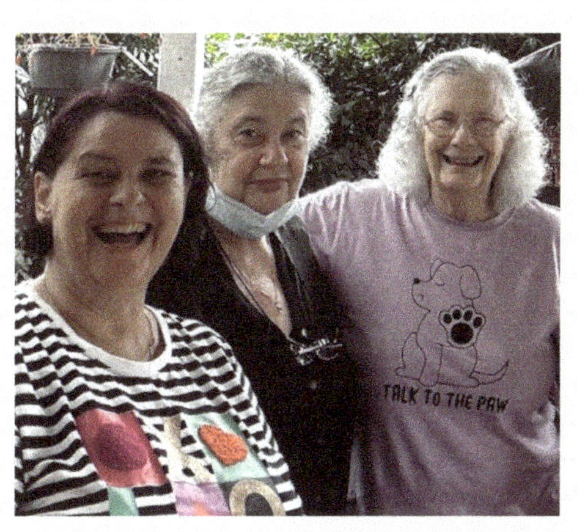

Me, Aunty K and Mum, April 17

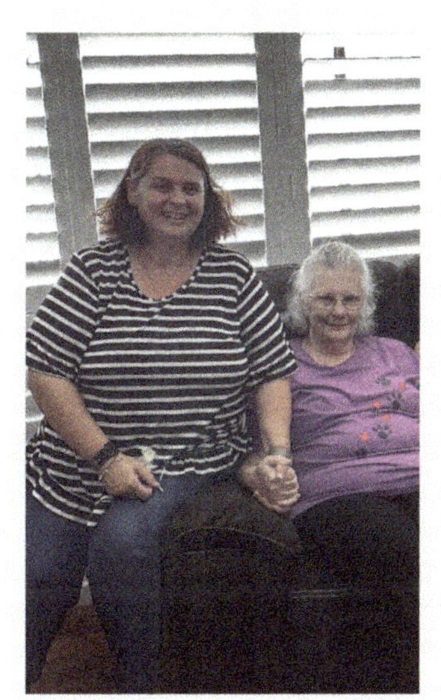

Making memories

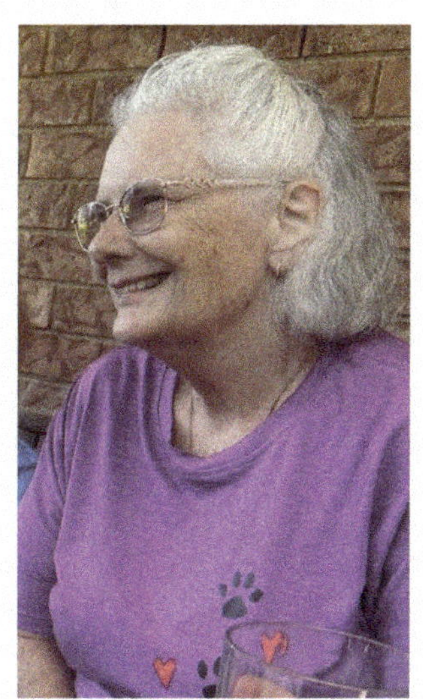

My beautiful mum at our last meal together

loving day. I took photos so I could remember this important time. Mum put so much effort into being well for this day, but at the end of it all she was spent.

The next morning after visitors left, Mum called me in. She was exhausted and said she was feeling very unwell. I took her temperature – she had a fever. I spoke with her about the options.

"We could go to the hospital and get treatment for whatever infection you may have, call the palliative care team for advice, take your oral antibiotics, or we could do nothing, but it's entirely up to you. From here on, Mum, the decisions are all up to you."

She shook her head *no* to all the options. "What's the point?" she said, adding, "I feel really sick. Is there something you can give me for that?"

"Of course, Mum. I'll get you something now."

I went out and got her a strong medication for nausea that the palliative care team had prescribed and left for her to take as needed. But it did nothing. After about an hour or so of fevers and feeling miserable, I asked her, "Do you mind if I call the palliative care nurse, Mum? I think we need more medication than I have to keep you comfortable."

"That's fine."

Her eyes were closed, there was a frown on her face, she was uncomfortable and just trying to hold it all together. I knew it was probably time to put in some little cannulas for the medications we would need over the next couple of days.

Unfortunately, Mum also understood what that meant. She opened her eyes, looked right at me and said, "Well, this is it then."

I just nodded. I had no words.

The palliative care nurses were amazing. They put in a pump and another little line just under the skin so I could administer the appropriate prescribed medications for pain and nausea as instructed. Within a few hours, Mum was struggling to stay awake. I was concerned she was becoming septic and the palliative care nurses seemed to share this concern. There was nothing left to do except sit with her and keep her comfortable. I gave her lots of hugs, I told her how much I loved her, how much I'd miss her. Aunty K and I realised we needed to move Mum to the special bed we had delivered as she started slipping in and out of consciousness. We got her up and, much to her distaste, put on a continence device so she wouldn't have to get up to use the toilet. We managed to safely manoeuvre her to the palliative care bed. Things were progressing fast. We let her know in one of her lucid moments that we should probably tell the others so they could come and see her.

"Is it really that time?" she said with disappointment in her voice.

I checked in with Aunty K and we both said, "Yes, we think it is," in unison.

Mum seemed uncomfortable with the idea of Nana sitting at her bedside. She thought it would be too stressful for a 94-year-old. Even on her deathbed, she was concerned about the welfare of others. She made us promise we would take care of Nana and not let her stay in distress for too long. We called and told them to come. Mum expressed how uncomfortable she felt in general about having people by her bedside upset. She didn't like the idea at all, but she was also aware of others' need to say goodbye.

Just before people arrived, Mum slipped into unconsciousness and never woke up again.

Her last words to me were, "I love you too."

It felt like she chose her time to leave on her own terms. I whispered to her, "You don't have to be awake anymore, Mum."

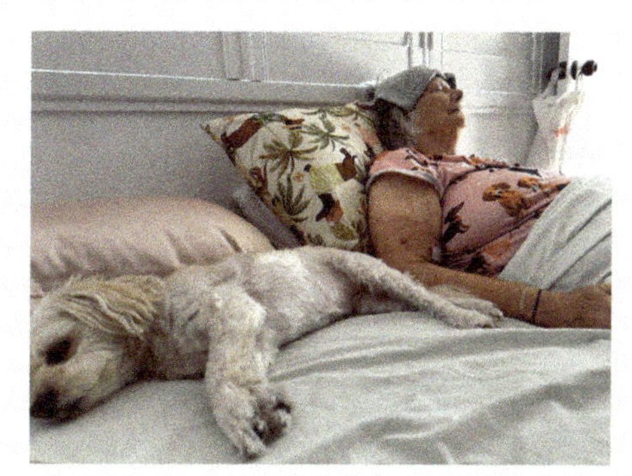

After visitors left, April 18 - Bella's vigil

It was sad I wouldn't get to speak to her again, but I was pleased she didn't have to experience the discomfort she was afraid of, quietly slipping into a sleep state instead. I propped Mum up and put the same little travel pillow I used for Dad around her neck, so she was more comfortable, and settled in for a long night. Nana and Nang stayed for a while until it became clear to me Nana was quite distressed. I felt she should probably go back to the motel to rest in line with Mum's wishes. I again felt it was appropriate to put on some background music to break up the sorrow and grief in the room, lightening things as I felt I knew Mum would have wanted.

That night and the next day seem like a blur of assessing for pain, trying to cool her down to reduce the discomfort from her raging fever, and interpreting which prescribed medication to administer as instructed. I was keen to keep my promise to Mum, ensuring she was comfortable and pain free. The palliative care nurses increased the dose of the background infusion in the middle of the day after her breakthrough medication requirements increased. Bella absolutely refused to leave her side. We occasionally picked her up and encouraged her to drink or go to the toilet. Aunty K was a constant source of support and care. I felt so relieved, both for Mum and myself, she was there. Being in my own home meant I was able to spend time with Benni every now and then, which was exactly what I needed. Just as we discussed, I brought the dogs in to see Mum at one point, so they knew what was happening.

Mum started to demonstrate some of the end-of-life breathing patterns, so I felt like it wouldn't be long before she passed. It was April 19 and my mum was in the final stages of dying. This felt excruciatingly hard. Having to do this a second time in such a short period was heart-wrenching. It was now just me, Aunty K and the dogs. There would be no more visitors and Mum stopped needing any more breakthrough medications. A calm came over the room. Aunty K and I decided to turn the music off and just spent those last precious hours telling her how much we loved her, holding her hand, tenderly washing and cooling her forehead, caring for her and Bella. It was the regulated, calm environment Mum expressed she wanted, and we were so grateful she could have the peaceful end-of-life care she requested. We had been taking it in turns leaving the room for a bit to get some rest, but just after 11pm her breathing changed again, and Aunty K and I agreed we should probably both stay in the room now.

At 11.15pm on April 19, 2025, three years to the day since we first saw the specialist in Brisbane, my beautiful mum passed peacefully in her home, surrounded by people who loved her and her beautiful Princess Bella. I turned off the pump as I had been instructed by the beautiful palliative care nurse.

Both Aunty K and I were quietly crying, and I whispered, "It's all over now, Mum."

Through my tears I heard a scratch at the door. It was Benni asking to come in to check on me. I gave her a huge hug through my tears and gently put her back in bed, amazed at her incredible intuitive timing. We pulled ourselves together and let the appropriate people know Mum had passed.

I made sure the dogs all got to say goodbye to her as promised. Bella stayed loyally by Mum's side until her last breath, just as Mum had wanted. Molly was in the room most of the time but we still made sure she got to say goodbye. When Benni and Freya came in to see her, you could sense their gentle knowing that Mum was gone. Freya wanted to get closer, so we let her give Mum one last lick on the cheek. Benni seemed to know she'd already left us and, while she looked at mum, she was more concerned about me and Aunty K. We flattened her bed, as we had been instructed by the palliative care nurses, and let the palliative care team know. We finally went to bed ourselves, but I don't believe anyone got any sleep. I was spent, devastated and when I crawled into bed with beautiful Benni and Freya all I wanted to do was hug them tight. *Mum was gone.*

A MOTHER'S LOVE

Mum, you taught me how to walk, talk and ride
From you I learnt about unconditional love and pride
You taught me how to spell, read and write
Then you watched me grow and dreamed about a future so bright
You taught me how to take the knocks in life with grace
Turn the other cheek, dust yourself off and get back in the race
You taught me how to bounce back after a big fall
Encouraged me to ignore those who would make me feel small
You taught me how much love a dog can bring into a home
Our shared love of dogs preventing us both from feeling alone
You taught me all about healthy relationships and how to forgive
Demonstrating the values by which you recommended I live
You taught me about strength in the face of hard times
Then you modelled forgiveness even to those who had been unkind
For now, I will live by my values, your wise words echoing in my head
I'm so pleased that before you were gone we left nothing unsaid
You taught me about honesty, trust and the value of helping another
I found my safe space in your company; I'm so
privileged to have called you my mother
You taught me so much in my life, but I still have so much to learn
For now, I will try to comprehend how, without you, the world will still turn

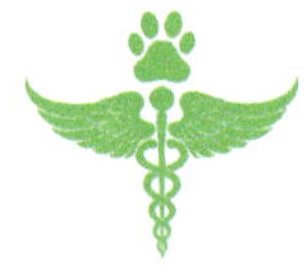

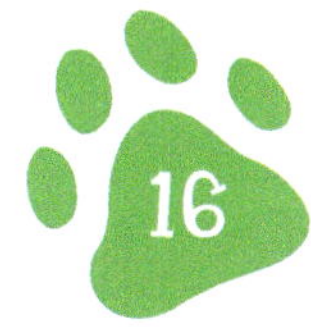

My beautiful Aunty K was a pillar of strength after Mum's death. She was respectful, caring, supportive and, most of all, embraced the same practice of prioritising peace. As per Mum's wishes, on May 31 at Benni's beach we held a lovely little service, scattering Mum's ashes to Celine Dion's *Because You Loved Me*. Those six weeks were harder than I expected but once her ashes were scattered I felt like she was finally at peace, which also gave me an enormous sense of relief. It felt so wrong having her in a box on the shelf. She lived such a rich and adventurous life, she needed to be free.

In the days after her death, my mother had one beautiful surprise for me. I received a call from a Buddhist nun from the palliative care charity Cittamani.

"Your mum asked me to call in case you wanted me to come and talk to you after she was gone. She thought you might need some support. Would that be okay?"

Mum knew I believed deeply in the Buddhist teachings and this last gesture of love and support took my breath away. I sobbed and gratefully agreed to meet with her. It was a nurturing and healing experience.

Two weeks after Mum passed, I also received a phone call from beautiful Ann Williams-Fitzgerald from Eagle Lodge. Before Mum died, I reconnected them so Mum could reminisce and perhaps find peace with her impending mortality. Ann was such a positive force in both our lives; I knew her wisdom and spiritual connection would help Mum through this difficult time. Mum had apparently asked Ann to call me after two weeks because that was traditionally when everyone goes back to their lives, and she thought I may be struggling by then. What a beautiful conversation and an amazing support from an old but true friend. To me, Mum truly embodied her values, showing compassion and modelling forgiveness, even to those who weren't kind to her, to her dying day. This remains my favourite thing about my mum. It's a value we shared and one I now vowed to continue for the rest of my life.

While grief frequently caught up with me in the months after Mum's death, having lost both my parents in such quick succession, I knew the importance of allowing grief to be present whenever it turned up. It felt important to give it space so I could effectively process it. Surprisingly, Nang has been a great source of support since my parents died. Her support with the practicalities involved in sorting through years of memories has been invaluable. We have laughed, reminisced and shared happy, sad and distressing memories of both Mum and Dad. I will always be grateful for her friendship in this time. I also promised Dad I would take care of Nang when he could no longer speak and his only way to communicate was joining our hands. I've kept my promise in every way I can, and continue to actively provide emotional and practical support to Nang whenever possible. I maintained contact with my amazing psychologist, without whom I would have struggled to make sense of it all. She has watched my transformation from acute, life-altering PTSD to stable PTSD, and gently guided me through it all with her wisdom and compassion. She's an inspiration to me, and I will be forever grateful for her support and professionalism in my lightest and darkest hours.

After Mum died, I went through her handbag to retrieve the identification documents Aunty K needed to complete her role as the executor of Mum's will. This was one of her specific instructions: "Make sure you give Aunty K all my identification."

Mum was always so organised. We used to make fun of her for packing weeks before a holiday. Death would be no different. She left specific instructions for us about her wishes regarding just about everything. Inside her handbag, I found several envelopes with handwritten letters penned in her last days to her loved ones. When the time came and I felt up to it, I was finally able to read my letter. It was like I could hear her voice from beyond. She was right back in the room with me, once again providing support and consoling me about her loss. She encouraged me to write the book you're reading now along with a children's book. I had been excitedly telling her I wanted to write a book for several years about Benni and her life as an assistance dog, and I had already named it *Being Benni*. Mum expressed how she wanted me to leave a legacy to immortalise the incredible dogs we had in our lives, how they helped us survive in the darkest of times. I made a quiet promise to her to do just that. She finished the letter with one line I will hold with me forever:

"... I love you beyond time, beyond life."

My mum was, and will continue to be, a positive force in my life. We didn't have the best start, and we had several years of estrangement in my early to mid-adulthood. I needed to mature and become an imperfect mum myself. I needed to develop the ability to see she was doing the best she could with the skills she had at the time, before I could finally have a healthy relationship with her. I'd like to say I regretted the delay in our connection, but I simply don't believe regret is a useful emotion. I prefer to appreciate the learning and growth we both gained from the challenges in our relationship. In many ways, those difficulties forged a deeper bond between us than we might have ever had without them. Our shared love of dogs, and experiences training our assistance dogs, Benni and Bella, brought us together, helping to heal some of the fractures in our relationship. I'm so grateful we found this peaceful place and sense of connection while she was alive with plenty of time to reap the rewards that this deep, restorative kind of relationship can bring to your life. I left nothing unsaid with Mum or Dad. I have no regrets and can truly appreciate and accept them warts and all, just as Mum had done for me after my PTSD diagnosis.

I believe it's an enormous privilege to care for someone during their dying days, and it was a great honour to do this for both of my parents.

This experience somehow went back into the depths of my soul and reshaped who I am as a person. Being able to offer compassion and care to someone who has hurt you so deeply, and being able to offer the same compassion and care to someone who has healed you so deeply, was profound and life-changing. Grief came with its gifts and curses, but I'll always feel grateful for ensuring my parents had a peaceful, pain-free end to their worldly experience. Even if this was the only reason I studied medicine all those years ago, it would have made it worthwhile.

The experience of caring for Mum and Dad while dying removed my fear of death, confirming to me there's a bigger picture and much more to existence than we think. However, one of the difficulties with this period of my life was the existential crisis that followed. *If the point of life is just to exist, and the source of all suffering is attachment, and you needed to stop attachment to stop suffering, then what's left? Why bother?* I've come to the realisation that not being attached is not the same as not caring. I wanted to end suffering for other people just like me. Being able to return to society as a functional support for others was a privilege not all people who suffered such a devastating change in life circumstances got to experience. Once I understood how the relationship with such an amazing animal could help rebuild your life after trauma, I felt a responsibility to share the information with others. We wouldn't just be helping humans. We would also be helping dogs, enriching their lives too.

Benni was, as always, a continuous source of both love and motivation throughout this time. Her presence always reminded me I need to consider both ends of the lead in all my training endeavours. With my newfound meaning and purpose, I was driven to complete what I started all those years ago – to become an accredited assistance dog training organisation in Queensland. I set about filling in all the paperwork and finally submitted my application, having competed my formal qualification as an assistance dog trainer.

I also kept my promise to Mum to find ways to immortalise these amazing dogs and the life-changing work they do every day through this book, the *Being Benni – Assistance Dog Benni* book and another children's book I wrote as a legacy just for Mum. The book *Being Benni – Bella is Sad* is a tribute to Benni's best friend, Bella, and the grief she experienced when her mum (and my mum) died. In a beautiful twist of fate, this book and both of the children's books were ready in time to be released in one big celebration.

THAT'S LIFE

Life is a journey full of twists and turns
A delicate tapestry woven tightly into your soul
No-one knows where this life might take you
It's a mystery, there's no choice but to accept

One morning is bright and full of dreams
The next can be dreary and full of dread
All things come to an end, good, bad and indifferent
There, in the midst of an ending, lies the spark of a new beginning

Only with hindsight is this new hope easily seen
Without clear vision, faith must guide you on your way
We're all interconnected, animals and humans alike, part of a bigger truth
To deny or harm each other is to deny or harm oneself

The healing you need may be right under your
nose, not in the form you think
The best medicine I ever took came not from a bottle but from a soul
The soul of a dog is so special and pure
Their love unconditional and their loyalty unsurpassed

Benni, you were the medicine I needed to heal
and integrate my broken parts
A renewed sense of purpose breathes life back into my heart
As you grow old and weary, your bones too sore to move on your own
I will take care of you, my beautiful Benni, a team to the very end!

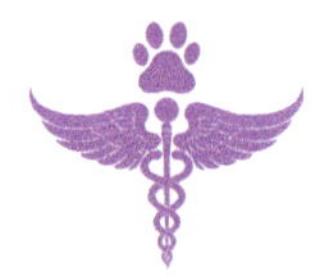

"We had a hell of a ride, didn't we?"

Dad was so right when he uttered those words. What a ride! Life has presented many challenges of which I'm proud to call myself a survivor. So much has happened since that fateful day in 2014, and these events have changed me in every way. Whenever something happened in my life, I always tried to make meaning of it, turning it into motivation or a catalyst for change of some sort. This was my pattern even as a child. I internalised the good, the bad and the ugly, and set about making meaning of it, then changing myself to be better, be smarter, be prettier, be *more* of whatever people said I wasn't enough of!

My life experiences have taught me what's on the outside, and therefore what others predominantly judge you on, is nothing more than packaging. I've been fat, skinny, extremely fit, extremely fat and all levels in between. I've been stupid, smart, extremely intelligent and all levels in between, but I was always the same me on the inside. At times, I was angry with people for judging me to be unintelligent or fat, or any other judgement they made, but I've come to understand this as a reflection of sorts. People don't judge you because of you. They judge you because of how *they* think, feel and behave themselves, all things you have no control over. I've learnt "the haters gonna hate", as Taylor Swift so eloquently puts it in her song *Shake It Off*.

People have asked me why I bothered with Dad. "Why not just cut him out of your life?" I've never believed in the cancel culture principal of cutting people off to heal. It just doesn't sit well with me to hurt someone to make the relationship easier on myself. Generally, while admittedly not the easiest option, I find maintaining healthy boundaries through difficult relationships far more healing.

Keeping discomfort at a distance heals nothing. Don't get me wrong. I do believe there are times when distance is required to keep you safe. This is often the case for very abusive relationships. However, the cancel culture ethos, I feel, is often used as justification for cases of discomfort or disagreement rather than abuse. Sometimes it seems people just want to be right or have the other person concede they were wrong. In my opinion, so much damage can be done to relationships when interactions are based on ego.

Difficult conversations are challenging, no doubt, but I feel they're a necessary part of all healthy relationships. People will always see things differently, as the lens we each perceive our reality through differs. I believe this is normal. In my view, you can grow up alongside someone, share the same circumstances and still walk away with entirely different interpretations of what happened. I've learnt respecting these differences is essential if you want to maintain healthy relationships.

Somewhere along the way, though, cutting people off became the default response to conflict and this goes against my values. To me, it overlooks the individuality of each person, their history and differing perspective, and ignores the potential harm that alienation can cause. The popularised practice of going "no contact" in the name of healthy boundaries might be well intentioned, but, in my view, it can inflict significant trauma, sometimes making you no better than the version of the person you're angry with.

I don't believe finding space and maintaining healthy boundaries requires villainising someone else. In my 40s, I told my dad I would never cut him off but I would also never chase him to have him in my life. I believe he didn't make much contact because it was of little benefit to him, but whenever I had contact with him it was nurturing for me instead of harmful. The freedom that comes from being able to hold your boundaries at the same time as holding compassion for the other person, and maintain whatever degree of contact this allows, is enormous. Regardless of how difficult a relationship is, I always let people know that even if I need a bit of space for a period, I will always be there on the other side of the difficulty, ready and available for healthy contact. Some people may prefer not to make contact and would rather keep distance than navigate difficult conversations. There is nothing wrong with this approach if that is what they can handle at the time. It's just not for me. I don't believe I could've healed my childhood trauma by cutting Dad out of my life altogether. The trauma simply would have sat there like a thorn in my side until he died, at which time I would have likely regretted never truly taking the time to understand and accept him for who he was.

I also experienced a lot of grief and upset in my life because the people around me didn't express love, compassion and support the way I expected them to when I was suffering. I've come to understand no-one else knows your subjective experience. They're often also traumatised with their own limited coping strategies or skills. We're all humans doing and behaving the best we can with the skills we have available to us at the time. I believe at some point in life you can no longer blame anyone else for your own behaviour, feelings or thoughts. Accepting responsibility, and not blaming someone else, doesn't mean I blame or punish myself. I just take radical responsibility for my own thoughts, emotions and behaviours.

When I began to understand that's all I ever had control over, it also freed me from a lifetime of feeling responsible for the thoughts, feelings and behaviours of others. Dad always said he was pleased he was so hard on me because it made me tougher. He also used to say he behaved the way he did because of how I made him feel – the classic "If you didn't do X, I wouldn't have needed to do Y to you."

If I'm responsible for my own thoughts, feelings and behaviours, then it follows others must be responsible for their own too! If I have no control over this then I also have no ability to change it. This stopped me from trying to change how others saw me. I knew my truth, which was all that mattered. This is a large part of why I feel such a sense of peace in life now. I hold myself very accountable for my own thoughts, emotions and behaviours, but this means when others even suggest I thought, felt or behaved in a way I'm certain I didn't, I no longer feel the need to defend myself.

Ultimately, I have come to accept people will believe what they want to believe, regardless of what I say. In my view, people's thoughts, emotions and behaviours are created within themselves, not by me. The peace that comes with letting go of the need to control the narrative is truly life-altering! Don't get me wrong. I hold no malice towards anyone who has misjudged me. I understand better than most how these misjudgements can form. These days, I try my best to love the way my dog does. I enjoy the precious moments I get to spend with those I love, and love unconditionally, while always holding my first and most precious value dear, my peace.

From counselling dog training clients, I have learnt the more attention you give to a behaviour, the more of that behaviour you will get. A lot of what we know about human behaviour and learning is based on studies, with questionable ethics by today's standards, done on dogs. It doesn't matter if you give positive or negative attention. Any attention has the potential to reinforce a behaviour. Conversely, the *less* attention you give to a behaviour, the less likely it is to be repeated. In my childhood this was all outside my control but, as an adult, I now apply this ethos to my human relationships as well. As adults, some say we teach people what behaviour and treatment we're prepared to accept. I believe my unrelenting standards, self-deprecating attitudes and general lack of self-care as an adult set the standard for those around me. Instead of being angry at someone else's behaviour or treatment of me, I now look at this as a form of communication.

Behaviour is essentially the external expression of a person's inner thoughts and feelings. If I feel someone's behaving badly, I now wonder what's going on for them instead of wondering what's wrong with me. Giving little or no attention to hurtful or unkind behaviours is what serves me best. I try to dedicate my time, love and respect to the people who offer love, support and care to myself and/or others. I hadn't realised it, but for most of my life I'd expended so much of my time and energy thinking about, stressing about and avoiding upsetting, unkind or difficult people around me. Very little of my time and energy were left to nurture the truly amazing relationships I was fortunate enough to have.

Upon reflection, I've realised misdirecting energy meant several important friendships were neglected. I've since made sure I nurture these important relationships as much as I can. This includes my amazing, lifelong best friend, Graeme Kay, whose friendship I will always cherish. His quirky sense of humour, intellectual banter and unconditional support throughout my adult life is something I'm deeply grateful for. I also feel I lost valuable time with my children through this misdirection of energy. I spent so much of my children's young lives working hard to prove my father wrong and, while this began with the noble intention of helping them with their homework, it ended in what felt like the complete destruction of my life and seemed to detrimentally affect all relationships within it.

I was very self-absorbed when I was sick, which I believe is a necessary part of the healing process, but it did blind me to the role I was playing in my own ongoing dysfunction. PTSD has a habit of decimating lives with symptoms like sleep disturbance, hypervigilance, loss of intimacy, lack of trust and numbing. These frequently, adversely affect close personal and intimate relationships. In hindsight, it's no surprise to me that so many of my personal relationships were affected and the resultant isolation further impaired my ability to make new relationships. If you want to fully heal, I believe the one person you absolutely must be honest with, and keep your promises to, is yourself! I have developed an understanding of how my thinking and coping styles contributed to the losses and dysfunction I experienced while unwell. I do everything I can to nurture the relationships that survived my PTSD diagnosis, while trying whatever I can to reconnect or at least hold compassion for the ones that didn't. Perfection is an illusion. We're all imperfect and will all make mistakes, which is why I believe strongly in forgiveness. I also believe it's important to extend yourself the same compassion and forgiveness you would give to someone you love. You only get one human in this life for whom you hold absolute lifelong responsibility – you!

Experiencing the stigma associated with having a mental health diagnosis came as a bit of a shock to me. I too have been guilty of using labels in the past (including narcissist) to describe difficult people in my life, which usually started with the intention of understanding them better. However, while useful in the short term, I believe labels can be very damaging. In my experience, labels don't just risk harming the person they're applied to. I've also come to believe they can make it easier for people to objectify and eventually dehumanise someone. Once you start to see someone through the lens of their label, it can become alarmingly easy to justify treating them badly. I'm very cautious about labels now and only ever use them to help me understand someone. Then I make a deliberate effort to set them aside. Every person is imperfect. We all struggle with something and so I prefer to offer compassion rather than judgement.

It was important for me to understand that I'm not my PTSD label and having a mental health diagnosis doesn't make me unstable or crazy. I also believe I would be no less of a person if I had any other form of mental health condition or personality disorder. I've undergone extensive investigations by experts and often joke that, unlike others, I know exactly what my mental health diagnosis is. I may have PTSD, but I also like to think I'm the only person I know who is *certifiably* sane! I no longer feel any need to defend myself and have stopped engaging in conversations about what alternative mental health condition someone else suggests I may have.

From my perspective, when people feel compelled to add or change a label, it usually reflects either a general lack of understanding or some kind of anger they're trying to express. I'm now also very grateful for my PTSD, having integrated this aspect of my reality into a healthy respect for the signals my body sends me to slow down or practise self-care. I'm unapologetically flawed, and frequently make mistakes for which I take ultimate responsibility, using them as an opportunity for growth. Embracing all parts of self, good and bad, past and present, is what forms the foundation for my internal peace.

It has always interested me how sometimes true strength appears to others (and even yourself at the time) as weakness. Sometimes, the most powerful lessons in life can come from your failures/weaknesses and not from your successes at all. Many of the people I knew when I was working as a doctor, earning a huge income, driving a nice car with the beautiful nuclear family and all the trimmings, commented how they thought I had it all together. When I stopped being able to function and lost everything, I appeared to have failed in every way.

People also told me how happy I looked when I was super fit and training for Ironman, yet this was one of the darkest times of my life. I have been to the bottom of the abyss and returned. I now like to think I can hold a torch, assisting others to find their own way out of their personal pit of despair. Bad things can happen to good people. Surviving them, and sharing the steps to thriving after disaster, has become a new focus in my life.

Some of the most incredibly successful people in life would tell you how it took several failed attempts to get to where they were. Failure is an integral part of success. Life is a perfectly imperfect series of experiences, good and bad, unique to the individual. When you realise only you can fully appreciate your individual life experience, it brings great peace. I think this peace is what Jack Palance's *City Slickers* character Curly might have been referring to when he stuck his index finger in the air and intimated that the secret to life was, "One thing. Just one thing."

I used to think happiness was a thing you searched for and eventually found if you were lucky enough. I spent many years in the search of this elusive thing they call happiness, much like Billy Crystal's *City Slickers* character Mitch. I certainly was very fortunate, but I wasn't at peace. In fact, there were many times when I was a long way from happy. I now understand happiness completely differently. The more I choose peace, the more I experience genuine happiness regardless of the surrounding circumstances or losses I may be experiencing at the time. For me, happiness is now a daily endeavour, and it depends on choosing peace.

My values are what define me, not my roles or my illnesses. The closer I live to my values, the more peace and therefore happiness I experience. When my functionality started to decline, I started to lose the roles I was used to playing. I was no longer a practising doctor, no longer the provider for the family, no longer financially secure, no longer a wife and no longer felt effective as a mum. I felt each one of these losses deeply and had to make a conscious effort daily to stop myself from getting utterly lost in them. I defined myself by the roles I played in the lives of others. These days, I no longer define myself by who or what I am to others or what I can do for people. I define myself by my values, which don't change like external definitions do. I value compassion for others even when they don't seem to have the same value for me, and this is partly because I don't see myself as separate anymore. What do I mean? This is one of the fundamental beliefs in Buddhism. We're all connected, so separation and therefore "self" is an illusion. We're all part of the same human/animal existence, and our welfare depends on how we treat each other and the Earth we survive off.

This may all seem a little esoteric on paper but, for me, this is now how I choose to live my life. I guess it's the ultimate form of integration. All of us are interconnected – humans, animals, plants, the Earth. The more we hurt or deny someone else's experience, the more we hurt ourselves. Having said that, as I said before, I also believe we're all equal and just doing the best we can with the skills we have available to us. I'm certain I wasn't a perfect doctor, wife or mother but I'm just as certain that I tried my best with the skills I had available to me at the time.

I now understand my illness and the aftermath impacted my entire family. I was broken and traumatised as a very young mum and, while I did heal from those wounds, I was still trying to prove something when my kids were little. I had been working so hard, and to lose functional capacity, lose status and deal with the irreparable damage to the family unit, which I thought would last a lifetime, felt unbearable.

Impermanence is another fundamental part of Buddhist philosophy. Happiness is transient but so is misery. All things will end, eventually! I enjoyed a lot of good times and laughs with my family and these are the memories I hold on to now. I've had to be honest with myself and accept that my behaviour was atrocious at times while I was sick and recovering. The people around me didn't behave the way I expected them to either when I was unwell, but who knows how you'll behave in any given set of circumstances? I wanted to be wrapped up in love and compassion but at the time it seemed like not everyone had the capacity to provide that for me. Despite how I felt, I firmly believe everyone did the best they could to navigate near impossible circumstances in what was an incredibly difficult and traumatic situation.

I don't feel like I behaved the way I would have liked either, often unfairly accusing others of being narcissistic or uncaring, projecting old wounds related to my father. It was an awful time, and I can only imagine the impact it had on those around me. My relationship didn't survive two years of that stress and although it was incredibly sad, if it didn't survive those two years, in my opinion, there was no way it would have survived the next eight. I believe things happen for a reason and I genuinely hope there's peace in the aftermath for all concerned.

In my opinion, you would be hard-pressed to find a job in this life more important than being a parent to your child. I was acutely aware of this and felt the responsibility of the role deeply. I wanted to be the best mum I could be and I did the absolute best I could with the tools I had, and worked on getting more tools when I felt those were inadequate. There was no criticism or standard you could throw at me that I hadn't already thrown at myself. I was always my own harshest critic, constantly reminding myself of my flaws and imperfections while striving to be a better mum. I was also holding those same harsh self-judgements, trying to become a better wife, a better doctor, striving to improve wherever I could as if there was nothing good in me unless I fixed it first. However, sometimes having the best of intentions isn't enough and I accept this may have been the case for me as a parent. It took a long time for me to stop trying to defend myself with, "I did the best I could." While I accept I did the best I could, I also feel I could have done better and didn't. This sad realisation nearly broke me.

Nothing had been more important to me than being a good mum but somehow, in the pursuit of providing the family with better opportunities, it seemed my intention was corrupted. The result was my downfall and the devastating aftermath. Acceptance was vital so I could take responsibility for my own behaviours, thoughts, emotions and choices. I couldn't change or regret the past. All I have is today. I now use every day as an opportunity to do, think and feel differently.

While I feel I was trying so desperately to do the right thing by my kids, by my husband, by society's and my own harsh standards, I forgot one of the other terribly important jobs I have in life; to care for the unique human I had been gifted with at birth, *me*. I always thought it was my job to care for others and someone else's job to care for me. Consequently, I frequently felt unlovable, isolated and alone when I realised they didn't care for me the way I cared for them. Unlike me, others didn't seem prepared to sacrifice their own welfare for mine and that always hurt deeply. Now I see this differently – maybe they just knew better! You see, by being so harsh on myself and only ever caring about my performance, as judged by and for others, I neglected to care for myself and this caused further harm through constant self-deprecation and unrealistic, unachievable goals.

Self-care isn't about preferring self over other. For me, it's about considering your needs equal to others. I believe this is the most profound gift you can give others, a version of you who also cares about your own needs. Setting the example for your loved ones to also practise self-care. I can hear my inner critic screaming at me. *How selfish can you be?* Looking after your mental, physical and emotional wellbeing isn't selfish. Only from a place of healing and genuine love can you be of service to another human being.

I now believe the best thing I can do for my relationships, for my work and for others is to be the most healed, peaceful, loving and compassionate version of myself I can be. I do wish I had known this when my children were young, but I can't regret what I didn't know. I always felt so privileged to be a mother and still do. I also felt privileged to be a doctor. When did it all become a chore instead of a privilege? I believe the turning point occurs when you start to pathologically self-sacrifice.

Neglecting your own needs for someone else's is an inevitability in life, particularly as a mum, and may be necessary for their survival at some point. However, I believe this has a limit in terms of both utility and survival, and somewhere along the way it becomes unhelpful for all parties. Benni reminds me every day about self-care and how important it is in the service of others. If I'm neglecting basic self-care needs like sleep, my mood will change and Benni, in her role as my assistance dog, picks up on this, alerting me. These behaviours (for example, bad moods) are a way my body communicates its unmet needs. This awareness can then be channelled into addressing the unmet need so I can be of more use to others. What use am I to anyone fatigued? My body spent years screaming out for my help and I persistently neglected it, until it decided it had enough. You can only ignore the signs for so long. If you don't listen or stop, your body or mind will do it for you. It's a lesson I learnt the very hard way!

I have always felt like I couldn't do the rocking chair regret thing, instead living life to its fullest whenever I could. As I got older, this morphed into a dislike for the word "regret", preferring to consider what the experience may have taught me instead, using it as an opportunity for growth. Developing PTSD had a devastating effect on all aspects of my life, including my relationships, but I may never have learnt so many things without that degree of hardship. Most importantly, I would never have met the beautiful Benni whose unconditional love and affection healed a part of me that may have remained wounded for life without her influence. If I'd walked a different path, I would never have become a dog behaviourist, may never have experienced the life-changing healing that a deep relationship with a dog can bring, and would never have found a job that fulfils my soul's purpose.

Benni also brought Mum and me together, providing me with an opportunity to experience a deeply restorative relationship. I got into medicine to help people but felt the medical profession was more geared towards *treating* people. I truly believe that what I do now *helps* people. At the end of each day, even the long ones, I leave work with a smile on my face, and in my heart, knowing I have contributed to the enrichment of the lives of both dogs and humans. My days are rich, purposeful, full of love and most of all peaceful.

Being able to return to function in society after my diagnosis with PTSD was an absolute privilege. I feel a deep sense of responsibility to raise awareness about mental health, reduce the associated stigma people are exposed to in the community and bring attention to the power of recovery through training an assistance dog. There have been so many times in the past eight years that Benni was my reason for getting out of bed and sometimes the only reason I survived the day. Training and caring for her gave me back my confidence, tested my frustration tolerance, increased my optimism, improved my self-efficacy and taught me how to function in my new reality. Her health challenges made me read medical literature again and forced me to cope with potentially life-threatening situations for her, proving my skills and knowledge were never lost. Her behavioural challenges, and my difficulties finding an appropriate trainer to meet her needs, also continually forced me to read and learn, which helped to heal my brain, to the point where I could again hope for a functional future.

I will be forever humbled by the process of training Benni. Just when you think you know it all and you're a great trainer, Benni introduces a new challenge. This has sparked in me an eternal curiosity and motivation to learn as much as I can about these beautiful animals, how they think and behave. This cycle of learning, from unconscious incompetence all the way through to conscious competence, is an ever-evolving process that keeps life interesting.

My dog taught me so much about safety in relationships. She taught me how special it is to just sit in discomfort with someone, no words, just being there. Sometimes when the world is a dark place to be in, you don't need advice or to talk. You just need someone to sit by your side while you navigate the dark by yourself. Benni also taught me about checking in when someone looks like they're struggling and, if they still don't look okay, to persist and just keep gently checking in.

Her amazing ability to look deeply into my soul, and see and accept me exactly as I am – fat, skinny, smart, challenged, wounded and brave – gave me strength. Her love is always unwavering no matter how crabby or difficult I am. Her trust in me made me more trustworthy and her unbelievable loyalty meant she never left my side, in good times and bad. There have been moments. I'm ashamed to say during the worst of my PTSD, I was impatient with Benni, bad tempered, annoyed and even at times yelled at her or tugged on her lead in anger. I feel shame for those times because I know if the tables were turned, she would show me nothing but patience and kindness instead. Even still, she accepted this flawed version of me, waiting patiently by my side until the healed, better version of me evolved. There's a reason DOG is GOD spelt backwards. Benni's appearance in my life was lifesaving, and my best description is heaven sent. Dogs are creatures that epitomise what I believe humanity means and I now strive to live more like my dog every day.

The prominent Swiss psychoanalytical psychiatrist Carl Gustav Jung once said,

"The privilege of a lifetime is to
become who you truly are."

While I finally feel like I'm at peace with who I am, can see a bright future, no longer feel the need to change myself to lessen the discomfort of others, and have achieved some happiness, life is unpredictable. If there's one thing that is certain in life, it's how new challenges are just around the corner! My new focus in life will be to use what I've learnt to shine a light from the edge of the abyss to help reduce suffering for others. I will strive to improve the relationship between dogs and their handlers, and reduce the stigma around mental health through the work I do in my business, Dogz 4 Life. At the time of writing this book, I have been personally training assistance dogs for over eight years and Dogz 4 Life has been helping people train their own dogs for assistance roles for five years. We will continue to provide evidence-based support to people with disabilities who wish to train their own dogs.

I hope the Dogz 4 Life *Being Benni* children's book series can provide some education for families around the roles of assistance and therapy dogs. And the *Being Benni – Bella is Sad* book will provide valuable, relatable support for children suffering the loss of a loved one or pet while also providing a legacy for my beautiful mum. Without my mum's love and support, even from beyond, none of this would have been possible. Benni has been, and continues to be, a constant source of inspiration, unconditional support and challenge to me. Her grace and support for both me and Bella after Mum's loss was so heartwarming to watch. Our training challenges still inspire me to become a better behaviourist, and to that end I have recently enrolled in a diploma of clinical animal behaviour (DipCAB – canine) through the Canine Behaviour College in the United Kingdom. I look forward to what the future holds and will be involving Benni in any future projects. When we leave this world, we hope to leave behind a legacy that will provide support and enrichment for many dogs and handlers after us.

One dog really can make a difference.
Benni truly was, and remains,
the best medicine for me!

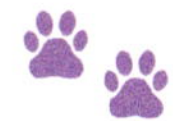

ACKNOWLEDGEMENTS

So many souls have been instrumental in my journey along the way and I'm bound to forget someone, so I would like to start with a general statement of thanks to all the wonderful people and creatures I met, worked with, studied with and befriended. I believe every experience, good and bad, can teach you something and I'm grateful for lessons both rewarding and difficult.

Baby Benni – I simply would not be here without your kindness, generosity of spirit, cheeky sense of humour and calming presence. You have taught me to be a better human and, in the process, how to speak dog. I love you more than I can express. I hope that you live a ridiculously long and happy life filled with love, treats and trips to Benni's Beach. You are my soul family so when you do leave this earth, I'm sure we will see each other again.

To my beautiful children, having you both remain the two best decisions I ever made. You were the drive to change and push through any barriers and limitations put in front of me to create a better future for you both. You have both grown up to be amazing, intelligent human beings, each successful in your own right in relationships, work and life in general. It's the greatest privilege of my life to be your mother and I wish you all the happiness, love, success and peace that life can bring.

To my wonderful mum who is no longer with us in this life, you remain my inspiration. I will forever be grateful for your sage advice, unconditional support and tenacious character. We didn't always see eye to eye but I always admired your courage. You suffered so much in this life but I believe your resilience and determination always shone brighter than your abusers and detractors. Because of you, I'm reminded daily that all it takes to survive is to get up one more time than you fall down. Benni, Freya, Bella and I miss you every day. I know you were worried about how Bella would cope once you were gone and she didn't have her "person". In accordance with your wishes I believe I've found a new handler for Bella so her work as an assistance dog will continue. She can have her new "person" and become an important part of their lives too. I know you will watch over her. This book and the *Being Benni* book series would never have happened without your support. Thank you for always being there, for your great advice, for your love and most of all for being my mum. If I had to choose again, I would pick you every time!

Dad, our personalities were so different we were bound to come to blows. I know you had a lot of hardship in your life. I hope wherever you are you can finally rest easy. I will always admire your fighting spirit and uncanny ability to see the finished product before a project even began. I kept my promise to look after Nang to the best of my ability. Thank you for giving me the gift of your acceptance before you departed this world. Looking after you in your last days was a privilege I will be forever grateful for. I know some of our most difficult times are penned in this book but I hope you can see it as a tribute to our ability to reach a place of mutual understanding and peace in the end.

Nang, thank you for the dedication and compassion you showed Dad in his last months on this earth. I'm grateful for your support and connection around Mum's death and in the aftermath of the loss of both my parents in such a short period of time. I know you're still grieving and I hope you can find some solace in the pages of this book. Dad lived a rich and interesting life and he shared many adventures with us all but none more than with you.

Lois, your unwavering belief in me at a time when I didn't even believe in myself was transformative. In my practice, I strive to be that person for my clients.

There were so many amazing, compassionate, caring junior and senior doctors who shaped my own development as a doctor and I will always be grateful for their support and wisdom. Without people like you, practising medicine would have been so much harder. Vivienne was one of these extraordinary doctors. I am so grateful for her presence in my life and her ongoing friendship despite circumstance and the distance between us. There were also some very difficult, entitled junior and senior medical staff from whom I learnt a lot about patience, understanding and navigating difficult people while still holding compassion for them. I'm grateful for both as they helped me to develop into the doctor and person that I wanted to become.

Kareem, your sense of humour, wit and intelligence got me through my intern year. Our time together was short but you had a huge impact on my life and our little family. Long after you had moved on, we told stories about your amazing energy and positive attitude. I was frequently reminded of your gentle irreverence for the pomp of the role and tried to propagate your infectious energy everywhere I went. Such fond memories, thank you!

Graeme Kay, my wonderful friend, I'm a bit lost for words. When we met, you were a teenager embarking on a whole new adventure, and I was a young mum finding her way in the world and healing from childhood scars. Our friendship has endured despite distance, busy lives, family commitments and differences. You taught me about true friendship, and I count myself extremely lucky to have this meaningful connection with another human being. Many people go through their whole lives without finding their "ride or die" and you, my friend, will always be mine. You're a constant source of inspiration, witty banter, weird philosophy and connection. May life treat you and your family with the respect, compassion and dignity that you afford others.

To my beautiful Aunty K. I'm so grateful to have you in my life. You're a constant source of strength and a guiding light. Thank you for putting up with my endless calls and texts in what has been a very difficult time. Mum was my North Star and I know you were hers. You're a wise soul and your sage advice is just what I need on those darker days.

Ann Williams-Fitzgerald, thank you for all your wisdom, advice and kind words. You came into my life at just the right time, and divine timing is something that has continued to be a feature of my life ever since. I thank you for your love and support over the years, and for reconnecting with Mum when she really needed you.

Bel, your support over the past few years has been invaluable. We share some parallels in experience but we also share strength of spirit, compassion and forgiveness as values. You're a special soul and my life has been enriched just knowing you.

Essa, my good friend, I'm so proud to have called you a friend. You're generous, kind, witty and funny. Most of all, you were my rock. In the darkest of times, you didn't run away from me. You ran towards me and for that I will always be grateful. I know God holds a special place for people like you, and up there, there's no more dips and trickles!

To all my nursing and midwifery family. Nurses and midwives are a special breed of human. These are the hardest working, kindest and most compassionate people I've ever met. I will always feel it was one of my greatest privileges to get to know you all and I miss our tearoom chats, dinners and hugs.

Ah, my friend Nele, working with you was so much fun! You brought a breath of fresh air to every day and it's an honour to call you my friend! You're an incredibly capable doctor, an amazing mum and all-round good human being. Thank you for your ongoing friendship and loving kindness over the many years we've known each other. Here's to many, many more!

Jo, my beautiful childhood best friend. Your warm smile always welcomed me and I was so grateful to have you by my side during what were the toughest years of my childhood. You are a truly amazing soul.

To my psychologist, your professionalism, support and occasional challenge has been pivotal in my recovery. Thank you for always making yourself available and in general for being the kind, warm, intelligent, regulated professional you are. The world is a better place because there are people like you in it!

Lisa, we met over dog grooming equipment but we became instant friends. Your kindness, support and love has been invaluable to me. I love you and all that you are, and look forward to many more years of spa days, trivia nights and friendship.

Shannon, thank you for always turning up. We haven't been friends for long but I feel like I've known you forever. I love our coffee days, catchups and chats. I hope we have many more in future.

Sam Gallagher, when I couldn't find a placement for love nor money, you were a beacon in the fog. Your compassion, kindness, care and willingness to take me under your wing was so refreshing. Thank you for your gentle support through some difficult losses and for trusting me to train dogs alongside you. The work you do is invaluable, and I appreciate you and your organisation more than you will ever know.

To Di, John (trainer) and the volunteers from In The Paws of Angels, thank you for accepting me into the fold. I feel like part of your little family and you have always made me feel welcome and supported. A special thanks for the hugs, Di – they always made my days a bit brighter.

Denise, my lovely friend, I feel blessed to have you in my life. Thank you for your support, care and understanding. I hope we can look forward to many years of friendship, joy, laughter and hopefully a few stage shows!

Roxanne McCarty O'Kane what can I say? I came to you with a nebulous plan to honour my Mum and the contribution our dogs have made to our lives. You nurtured and supported me through what was a very difficult but incredibly healing journey. You walked with me through the difficulty providing much-needed encouragement and support. You are a truly gifted, patient, kind and inspirational human being. I believe powers greater than the two of us bought us together and I will be forever grateful. Thank you from the bottom of my soul. I will always appreciate you!

ABOUT THE AUTHOR

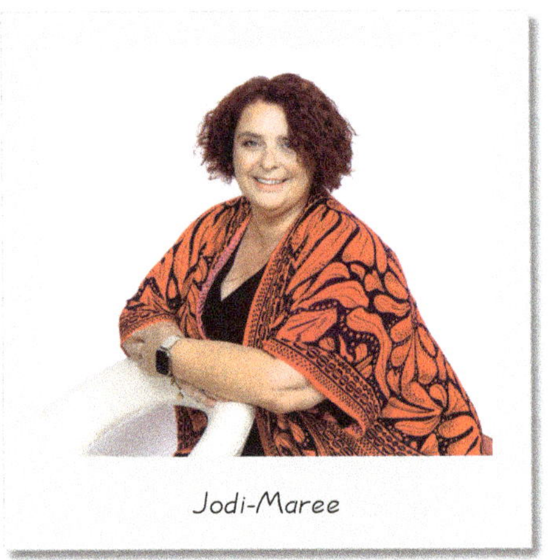
Jodi-Maree

Jodi-Maree Cronin is the director of Dogz 4 Life Pty Ltd and the founder of Canine Integrative Relational Therapy. Her qualifications include: MBBS, B Biomed Sci, clinical Cert CCPT, Dip Counselling, Cert IV in Animal Behaviour and Assistance Dog Training, Cert III in Companion Animal Services, and Student DipCAB (Clinical Animal Behaviour – Canine) through Canine Behaviour College UK.

Jodi is a retired doctor, medical manager and adult educator who has dedicated her adult life to the service of others. Throughout her working life, she has strived to be up to date, knowledgeable, approachable and understanding of differing perspectives. After working for many years in high-pressure environments, she's aware of the demands and challenges of being a working parent, professional and partner, as well as the impact this can have on your health and wellbeing, and now enjoys a simpler life.

After retiring from medicine, Jodi has spent the last eight years training assistance animals for individuals with life challenges, witnessing firsthand the power of the human-animal bond. This, combined with her desire to help others, commitment to excellence and interest in animal welfare, guides both her dog training and animal-assisted therapy practice.

Her professional development courses bring together her expertise in human health and behaviour, animal behaviour and training in an empathetic, evidence-based approach unique to Dogz 4 Life.

With a novel perspective shaped by her life experiences and extensive background in adult education, combined with proven public speaking skills, she is also available for practice supervision (including critical incident debriefing), as well as public speaking engagements by arrangement.

https://dogz4life.com.au

ABOUT THE CO-AUTHOR

Beautiful Benni is a German Short Haired Pointer and underwear thief. She's a trained, now retired, assistance dog that helps other dogs in training. Born in 2017, she loves treats and walks on the beach.

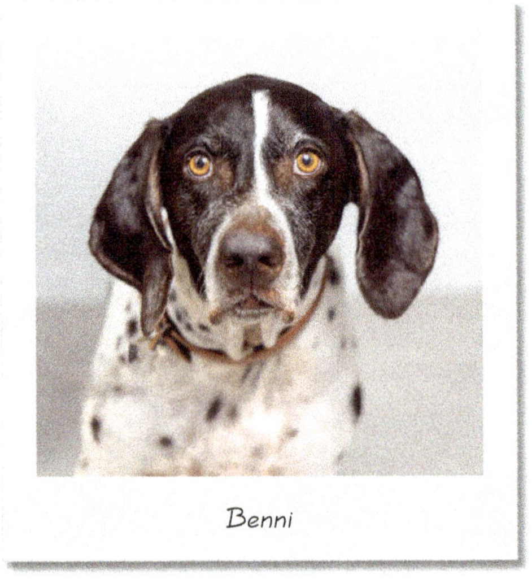
Benni

OTHER BOOKS FROM DR JODI-MAREE CRONIN

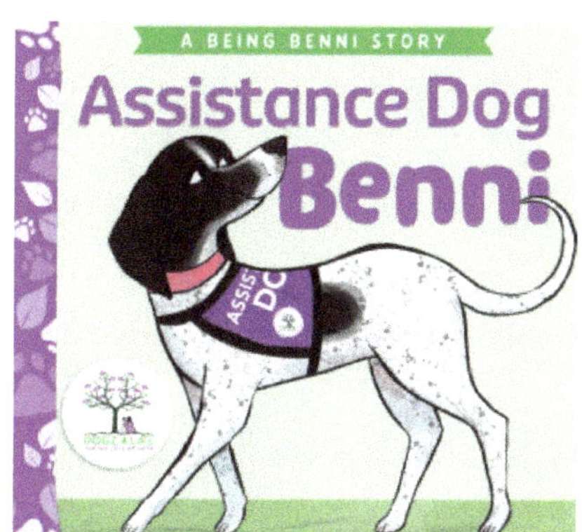

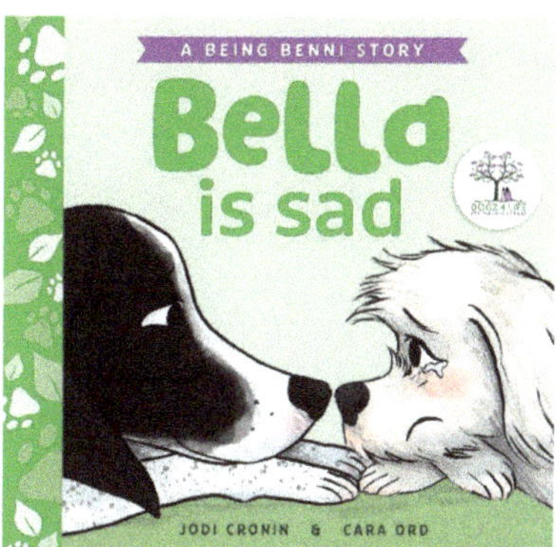

Discover the Being Benni series at

https://dogz4life.com.au/shop/

REFERENCES

1. Cate Swannell, "Mental health: Why doctors don't seek help," InSight, Issue 24, 27 June 2022. Retrieved on 10 November 2025 from https://insightplus.mja.com.au/2022/24/mental-health-why-doctors-dont-seek-help/
2. Claudia Zimmermann, Susanne Strohmaier, Harald Herkner, Thomas Niederkrotenthaler and Eva Schernhammer, "Suicide rates among physicians compared with the general population in studies from 20 countries: gender stratified systematic review and meta-analysis," The BMJ, 10 June 2024. Retrieved on 10 November 2025 from https://www.bmj.com/content/386/bmj-2023-078964
3. Pranjal Malewar, "Landmark study reveals cell-level brain changes tied to PTSD," New Atlas, 6 July 2025. Retrieved on 11 November 2025 from https://newatlas.com/mental-health/landmark-study-reveals-cell-level-brain-changes-tied-to-ptsd/
4. Phil Joyce, Charlotte Sills, "Skills in Gestalt Counselling & Psychotherapy," Sage, April 2018. Fourth edition. Retrieved on 10 November 2025 from https://uk.sagepub.com/en-gb/eur/skills-in-gestalt-counselling-psychotherapy/book253923
5. Öner Özdemir, Gökçe Kasımoğlu, Ayşegül Bak, Hüseyin Sütlüoğlu and Süreyya Savaşan, "Mast cell activation syndrome: An up-to-date review of literature," National Library of Medicine, 9 June 2024; 13(2). Retrieved on 10 November 2025 from https://pmc.ncbi.nlm.nih.gov/articles/PMC11212760/
6. Phil Joyce, Charlotte Sills, "Skills in Gestalt Counselling & Psychotherapy," Sage, April 2018. Fourth edition. Retrieved on 10 November 2025 from https://uk.sagepub.com/en-gb/eur/skills-in-gestalt-counselling-psychotherapy/book253923
7. Meg Kirby, AAPI Training Manual. The Equine Psychotherapy Institute, 2022.
8. Phil Joyce, Charlotte Sills, "Skills in Gestalt Counselling & Psychotherapy," Sage, April 2018. Fourth edition. Retrieved on 10 November 2025 from https://uk.sagepub.com/en-gb/eur/skills-in-gestalt-counselling-psychotherapy/book253923

www.ingramcontent.com/pod-product-compliance
Ingram Content Group UK Ltd.
Pitfield, Milton Keynes, MK11 3LW, UK
UKHW062303290726
14090UKWH00017B/854

9 781764 372428